I0410298

She Will Always Carry On

How I Beat Cancer Against All Odds

by
Maddy Ritchie

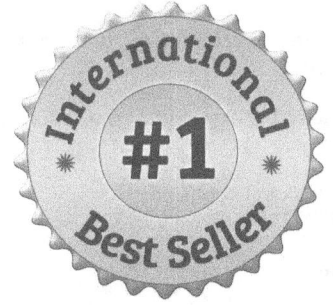

Amazon #1 Best Selling Book
in 4 Countries and 17 Categories
Ranked #155 Amazon.com.au

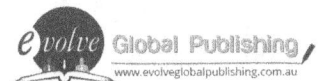
evolve Global Publishing
www.evolveglobalpublishing.com.au

COPYRIGHT

Copyright © 2016 by Maddy Ritchie

All rights reserved. No part of this publication may be reproduced, distributed or transmitted in any form or by any means, including via photocopying, recording, or other electronic or mechanical methods, without the prior written permission of the publisher, except in the case of brief quotations embodied in critical reviews and certain other noncommercial uses permitted by copyright law. For permission requests, write to the publisher, addressed: "Attention: Permissions Coordinator", at the address below:

Limit of Liability Disclaimer: The information contained in this book is for information purposes only, and may not apply to your situation. The author, publisher, distributor, and provider provide no warranty about the content or accuracy of content enclosed. Information provided is subjective. Keep this in mind when reviewing this guide.

Although the author and publisher have made every effort to ensure that the information in this book was correct at press time, the author and publisher do not assume and hereby disclaim any liability to any party for any loss, damage, or disruption caused by errors or omissions, whether such errors or omissions result from negligence, accident, or any other cause.

Website: www.maddyritchieauthor.com

Social Media:

LinkedIn: https://www.linkedin.com/in/maddyritchie
Facebook: https://www.facebook.com/maddyritchieauthor
Twitter: https://twitter.com/maddyritchiee

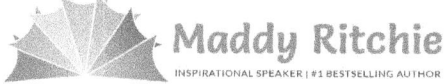

Maddy Ritchie
INSPIRATIONAL SPEAKER | #1 BESTSELLING AUTHOR

Ordering Information: Quantity sales. Special discounts are available on multiple purchases by corporations, associations, and others.

For details, contact the "Special Sales Department" at the address above.

--1st edition, 2016
First Published 2016 for by Evolve Global Publishing
PO Box 327 Stanhope Gardens NSW 2768
info@evolveglobalpublishing.com
www.evolveglobalpublishing.com

Book Layout: © 2016 Evolve Global Publishing

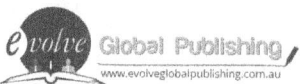
www.evolveglobalpublishing.com.au

ISBN: (Paperback): 978-1-63587-654-3
ISBN: (Hardcover): 978-1-63587-659-8
ISBN-13: (Createspace): 978-1541085022
ISBN-10: (Createspace): 1541085027
ISBN: (Smashwords): 9781370982103
ASIN: (Amazon Kindle): B01MSP86MJ

This book is available on Barnes & Noble, Kobo, Apple iBooks (digital), Google Books (digital)

Table of Contents

*This book is dedicated to the children who
lost their battle to childhood cancer.*

I live for you.

*Many thanks to Michael Crossland and
Andrew Hellmich from Impact Images.*

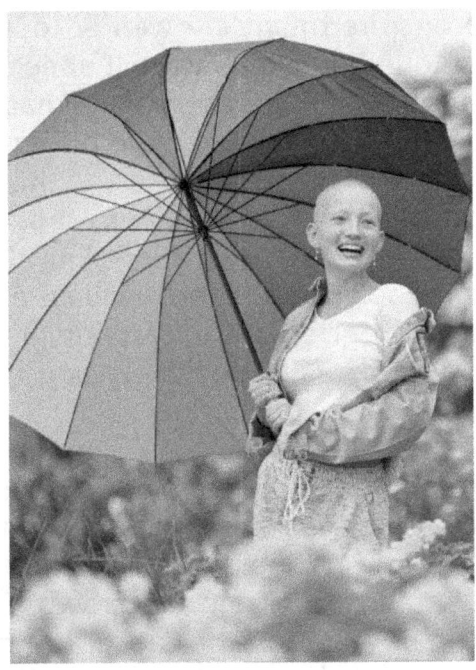

ABOUT THE AUTHOR

At the age of 17, only a week out from graduating from high school Maddy Ritchie was diagnosed with a rare childhood cancer called Rhabdomyosarcoma. She was given most likely three months to live and had to undergo 12 months of the most enduring and intense treatment regime to have some sort of chance at life. Through her horrific adversity, she found hope and healing through writing, she is raw and real when it comes to the truth of cancer on the individual and the others that surround them. A young girl who was self-conscious, lacked a sense of purpose, very materialism and took many things for granted had her world turn upside down when she was diagnosed with cancer. It changed her as a person forever but for a good reason.

Her determination inspired many, she wanted to share her personal story with the world in hopes people will understand, relate and be more aware of the real issues and stigma that surround cancer in today's society. She found through the power of her mind and within herself that she serves a purpose and that she can recover even when the odds were so against her. Maddy Ritchie is a #1 international bestselling author of "She Will Always Carry On". Maddy writes about the good and the bad days of her experience, how to cope with such grief and uncertainty, relationships, and how to look at your adversity positively and the power of the mind!

Maddy is an inspirational and engaging Speaker on overcoming extreme adversities. Her openness with her personal life, what she faces every day and her passion for making a change in the world is one that stands out from the crowd. She talks openly about her pain, the devastation the cancer left on her body, the lack of funding, the inequalites in attention which certain cancers get today, and that even through horrific times, we all can make it through by sheer determination and will power.

Chapter One
The Beginning

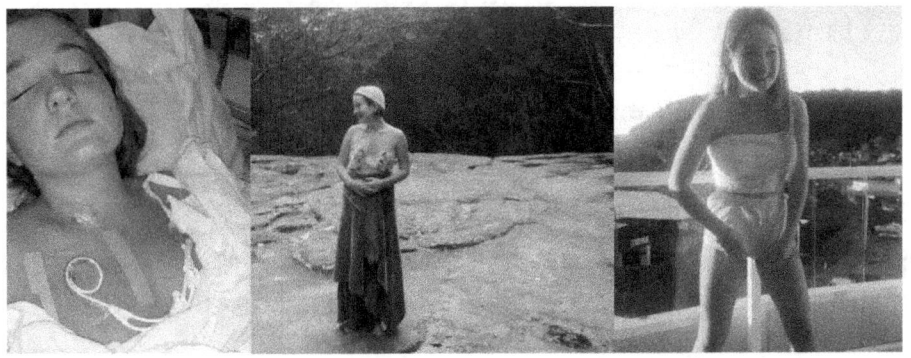

Cancer. A word I was definitely aware of but never understood.

It's in old people right or genetically passed on in families....

I wanted to write this book as I found a lot of people don't realise the reality and pain somene with cancer goes through every day and the impact it has on their family. There needs to be more education and awareness in communities and societies about the types of cancers, treatment, prevention and warning signs. We hear more about breast and bowel cancer but little about childhood cancers. I would love all cancers to be just as important....

In the month of October 2015 on a beautiful spring day, life as I knew it completely changed and I guess I felt it was stolen from me. The word cancer became my reality, and my fight for survival had just begun.

I had just graduated from high school in the last week of September. I had struggled immensely with my high school life. I had moved high school four times. I was at an all Girls' school, Performing Arts school, Christian school and a public school. I pretty much experienced every kind of school on offer. I never felt completely comfortable at school and never felt that I fitted in. To be finishing school was so exciting for me and all I wanted to do was to explore the world and travel.

June 2016 was to be an exciting year as I was saving money to travel to Spain. I have to be honest I didn't study that hard for the HSC exams; I'd just do my best. I always felt it wasn't going to determine my future.

Throughout 2015, I was struggling a lot with my energy levels. I was always tired and felt run down. I never really understood why. My doctor and my mum thought I was anaemic. I took iron tablets and started eating more red meat. Mum thought that with school, assessments, social life and the monthly women's thing I was over doing it but I was just doing what every 17-year old does.

The first sign that something was not right was my left butt cheek would ache uncontrollably. I would be sitting down, and within five minutes it would ache and become very sore. At the time I thought it was a little strange and just thought maybe I'm sitting too much... Really Maddy Really!!??

A few days later I noticed a little lump pushing out of my left groin along my bikini line. It felt rock hard. I showed my mum and she organised for me to see a lady doctor. My mum thought the most likely outcome was an ingrown hair from shaving and that I may need cream or antibiotics. I was still going about my daily life, studying, going to the beach and working at the local Café Restaurant as a waitress.

I saw the local doctor about the lump and she seemed unsure and thought it was probably an ingrown hair too and gave me a script for antibiotics. Looking back now at this moment makes me angry. I felt that with these doctors' qualifications, having spent years studying at University or College should have had more knowledge in knowing that this lump was definitely not from an ingrown hair. It makes you lose trust in the people that you should be able to trust. It's something that dearly bothers me and still does today.

Those matters of weeks could have been the difference between life and death and changed the course of my treatment and the severity of my cancer.

I remember walking out of the doctor and thinking what a relief; I'll be fine, little did I know what was to come.

The October long weekend I had prepared to go to my good friend Emily. It was going to be hot, and we decided to make it a beach and catch up time. I remember the first night at Em's house, I was getting changed in front of the mirror, and as I looked up, I saw that the lump on my groin had doubled in size. The colour of my skin in and around the lump was purple and yellow. Still I didn't freak out, nor did I honestly worry that much.

While I'm now writing this, I wish I could scream and yell at myself back then as these were the warning signs. To this day, I still beat myself up about it and wished I'd have done something straight away. It was there, it was right in front of me! The devil inside!

The next day we walked to the beach as we were planning on meeting another good friend Hephzibah. The walk was no more than 1km up the road; halfway there I was completely out of breath, and my legs were sore. I was so embarrassed by this; I hid it from Emily and just thought I was terribly unfit. When we arrived at the beach, I felt like I had just walked 10km. Whilst sunbathing I noticed immediately how bloated my stomach was. Later that night I began to think something was wrong. I seemed to feel weaker and out of breath. The bloating in my stomach and severe aches in my left butt cheek concerned me, and the lump had become purple. Little did I know that in these moments, my body was loosing, I was dying slowly...

That next morning I panicked and called my mum. It was that morning that my instinct and my consciousness began to tell me "Maddy something is wrong, get help ASAP".

That afternoon my mum took me straight to emergency at Gosford Hospital. We saw two different doctors; they decided to do a blood test and recommended an ultrasound the next day. I still didn't know what was happening to my body and it was killing me inside. My heart and consciousness were telling me to act fast, but I couldn't do anything more to speed things up, it really upset me. I just wanted to know what this THING was.

The next day I went to the pathology clinic for my ultrasound. The radiologist began to go over the lump and on the screen it was the oddest-looking thing I had ever seen. It looked like a black ball, more like the size of a small fist. At that moment looking at the screen, I knew I had something bad, real bad. The idea of cancer still hadn't crossed my mind. Even the radiologist seemed a little unsure. He had another radiographer have a look also. They both agreed I should have a biopsy as soon as possible.

Well that was just great, walking out for a second time with no real answer although I knew something bad was happening inside of me.

My mum worked at the SAN Hospital in Wahroonga as a booking clerk. She had been there for 8 1/2 years and knew a lot of surgeons and specialists. The next day she took my ultrasound report to her workplace and sent it to Dr Parasyn who is a General Surgeon at the SAN, Randwick Children's Hospital and Westmead Hospital. Within two hours my mum received an urgent call from Dr Parasyn. He organised a biopsy for the next morning.

My mum called me immediately and told me what he had said. I could tell in mum's voice she was upset and very worried. We still talked about it being a cyst, inflammation or abnormal growth.

Friday the 9th of October, is a day I will never forget. A day that will always stay with me for the rest of my life. I was due for my biopsy at 9am, and my results was to be ready by 4:30pm.

The biopsy was very uncomfortable. They had numbed the area, but I could still feel the needle inside of me. I could watch as the needle went straight into the middle of lump to take tissue out. I couldn't help but notice how the doctor and nurses in the room were very silent during it all.

I went off to the local shopping centre, and mum went back to work. I had only been there for a couple of hours when mum called me sounding very distressed. She had gotten a call from Dr Parasyn, and he wanted to see us right away. Sitting on the bus back to the hospital felt like the slowest bus trip ever. My impatience and my eagerness to know were getting to me.

My head and my heart began to tell me it was cancer. I had heard of lumps and tumours before that turned out to be cancerous. I clenched my body, with much sorrow and despair. I was telling my body "I'm sorry" over and over again, sounds crazy but I didn't listen to the signs and signals of something is wrong. It was all there, but I chose to ignore it. Everything began to finally fall in its place and make sense. I had no doubt that the results would be cancer. I just knew by this stage... FINALLY.

Once off the bus, I ran into the hospital and up the stairs. I had reached the corridor before I almost collapsed. I threw my body up against the wall stumbling to find my water bottle in my bag. I was completely out of breath, with my heart racing and my head thumping. I finally found my water bottle, and within seconds I downed more than half a litre of water. It took me a good minute to get myself back together. My body was deteriorating; I was struggling to breathe just by running through a corridor and up a set of stairs...

Mum was waiting for me outside the clinic and showed no sign of panic. She now says that her insides were all over the place, but she wanted to stay strong for me. Shortly, Dr Parasyn called us in.

He was a very lovely, warm person; he seemed almost excited to see me. We all sat down, and he asked me about how I was going and our family history health wise. He asked to see the lump, so I lay down on the bed. I noticed when he saw the lump his mood changed, he seemed very quiet.

He sat me down and the first thing he said was "Maddy you are terribly out of breath and very very tired under your eyes, how long have you felt like this?" Neither of those two observations were a surprise to me at all, I said: "probably within the last month or so I started noticing I was weak and tired especially doing anything physically hard and I sometimes struggled to breathe".

He typed away on his computer what I was saying, he then turned to me in a very stuttered voice with a face filled with shock and said "I'm so sorry Maddy we found Blue Cell cancer tissues in the lump, you have cancer of the pelvis. We still can't determine what type of cancer or what stage but you have CANCER; I'm very sorry"

My mum let out an immediate outcry of "WHAT!?"

I remembered I just stared at the white blank wall ahead of me, I didn't feel anything. I didn't even shed a tear.

Because the pathology tests weren't fully finished, he would have to call my mum on Monday to explain what is next. We left for home. The drive home was silent, mum and I didn't talk too much. I had put my earphones in and my mum listened to the radio.

I could see that my mum was crying through her sunglasses. That weekend, I didn't mention it to anyone nor did I talk about it much. I kind of went on for those two days pretending that nothing was said to me. I noticed I got worst though, I couldn't move from my bed and I felt very light headed and almost kept collapsing.

I didn't go into work because I felt so sick. That weekend seemed to drag forever. It was so difficult waiting. I went back to school to sit my first exam which was music theory on the Monday and mum went to work. I wasn't even sure half the time what I was writing down, I had to keep it together. It only went for an hour, and I immediately left not even saying goodbye to anybody and ran to the closest toilets. I vomited, my eyes rolling through my head and pretty much collapsed on the cold hard ground. I have never told anybody about this incident until now.

Mum told me it was terrible waiting all day for Dr Parasyn to ring. Finally at 4pm, he called my mum and said we needed to be at Randwick Children's Hospital first thing Wednesday morning for scans, tests and to meet with Paediatric & Adolescent Oncologist, Dr Antoinette Anazodo and her team. We have to get onto this as soon as possible; we don't know what the cancer is doing or how fast it could be potentially growing.

I felt numb, I just didn't understand... how? Why????

I also didn't realise the extent of how bad the cancer was, but I was soon to find out.

I still didn't know what was to come, nor did I understand or know what I was about to go through. I was okay about it... WHY WOULD ANYONE BE OKAY ABOUT GETTING CANCER!? I still don't fucking know to this day, but I was so unaware nor did I know of the brutal pain that was set in stone in front of me. I guess you could say I was just really uneducated and didn't know the reality of what was to come.

I could not sleep that night. My mind was going nuts the whole night long, it couldn't be put to rest. I was thinking of all the things I would have to do to rid myself of this cancerous lump.

Surgery...?

Chemotherapy...?

What else?

I had read up a lot about conspiracies, about the government and the world before my diagnosis. I had lead myself to believe that chemotherapy doesn't work, more people die than live from being treated this way or suffer long-term consequences. It was a way for population control, money and greed. I wasn't a full believer of this though, as a lot of my sources of information weren't always reliable.

I was overthinking like crazy, and I grabbed my phone to look up alternatives such as cannabis oil, gene mutation or travelling to Europe to get these special treatments that have a fighting chance. I looked at this for hours that night, yet I still hadn't been given my diagnosis or treatment plan...

Wednesday morning finally came, my appointment wasn't until 2pm and time seemed to stand still and go so slow. The drive to Randwick is at least a good hour and a half. My mum drove me, and we were to meet my father at the hospital.

My parents had only briefly seen each other earlier in the year when I had my tonsils out. They had been divorced for a couple of years. They seemed to be only centred on me and told me so.

I also hadn't seen my father in a long time either, we had a falling out and with his job he was away a lot. Our relationship over the last couple of months has been rekindled, and he now lives on the Central Coast with his partner.

We found our away to the Children's hospital and made it to the waiting room. I knew it would be at least another 24-48hrs to fully have a clear idea of what my cancer is. We met with Dr Anazodo.

A very nice, strong lady who knew her stuff.

She was asking me many questions about my health in the past 12 months, and I explained all my signs and symptoms and also the fact that within the past three days I had deteriorated more and more. She was very troubled by this. Dr Anazodo was very straight forward and explained that I have some sort of childhood cancer. The most likely outcome of my cancer is between Lymphoma and Leukaemia and explained that the cancer must be growing very fast and rapid due to the deterioration of my body within the last few days.

We only had the biopsy results and needed scans to determine the type of cancer and stage.

Dr Anazodo had a look at the lump, and as I laid down and showed her, I noticed her eyebrows rose up. I myself noticed that this time the left side of my pelvis/stomach area began to grow more and more discoloured. The lump itself was like a huge rock under my skin.

As she was softly pushing down on the lump, I felt like vomiting. It was beyond uncomfortable.

Dr Anazodo ordered scans to be done. The scans would be classified as an emergency and results within 24 hours. I was to have an MRI, CT, and PET scan. All of which are different, longer and show different ways of looking at this tumour to determine the final result. I was also to be admitted into the hospital and expected to stay for a few days.

Dr Anazodo needed to leave due to a meeting, so she called in her registrar and a few of the nurses on her team. The registrar wanted to look over me to get an idea of my blood pressure, heart rate and the impact the lump was having on my body. My heart rate was up, my blood pressure was low. I showed signs of much weakness in my upper body and legs.

My body was also uncontrollably aching everywhere.

The registrar explained that I would be having an MRI, then CT scan and later that night a PET scan. At the time I had no idea what any of these scans even were, what they do or show.

It was now that I began to feel afraid yet I was so powerless to stop it or do anything to help the situation that I was in. I began to cry uncontrollably. The registrar calmed me down.

To add to everything I was to have a cannula put in my arm. A cannula is a temporary needle that goes into one of your veins providing fluid, antibiotics or contrast into your body. I needed it mainly for the CT and PET scan.

I have a phobia of cannulas, they hurt like crazy when putting it in, and they're just not nice. Usually you can have numbing cream put on the area, but there was no time for this. I became deeply upset; it hurt like hell and was just the icing on the cake to everything else going on. Mum ran into the room and began to calm me down.

As the nurse began looking at my right arm for a vein close to the skin's surface, I braced myself; as she inserted the needle I screamed my head off; I think I screamed out the whole hospital.

After calming down I was taken into a room with four beds, three of them already occupied with children who had obviously been in for surgery. My first thought was "are you're kidding me? I have just been diagnosed with cancer and your putting me with other little kids under 10 years old in a room that I'm expected to stay in for a few days...!?!?!" I later learnt that they were real busy and had no other room, so I quickly moved past that thought and sucked it up.

They did my height, weight and took my blood pressure and temperature.

I noticed I put on even more weight again by this time... by this stage, I was pushing nearly 57kilos! When only a month ago I weighed about 52, this was alarming. I hadn't eaten McDonald's for the past month every day... I was very confused. I later learnt that it was due to my cancer. Since then I have always told a lot of people that putting on a significant amount of weight, becoming very bloated suddenly when you're leading a fairly healthy lifestyle is a sign of a potential cancer. A lot of symptoms of cancer can be shown through significant weight gain; 98% of people I have told this too had no idea.

As I sit patiently watching the TV in my hospital bed, dad sitting in the chair beside me, my mum was pacing around back and forth looking very lost and utterly confused with everything that was happening I couldn't help but think how she was trying to stay strong; although I noticed she would go away and come back looking very teary.

It was nearly 6pm, when a nurse and wardsman came to the end of my bed to tell me I was going for an MRI scan. The scan goes for 40 minutes, and I had to drink this weird tasting contrast drink beforehand. Once in there I thought about my whole life; I had the same thoughts every time I had a scan. You look back on your life and wonder where did it all go so horribly wrong? And then you start to overthink... regrets fill your mind, a lot of anger too. My head would curse and scream these thoughts and say such things as "fuck you God, how dare you; you're not there; nothing is there, all religion is bullshit" or "whoa life is so shit, might as well die now if this is my life"...

It was 11pm by the time I got back to the ward and finally completed all three gruelling scans. Both my parents eagerly waiting, yet they were so tired. I told them to go home; they promised me they would be back first thing in the morning.

I slept like a baby all night as I think I was physically and mentally exhausted.

I woke up the next morning filled with... well I wouldn't say excitement, but I was just eager and keen to know what was happening in my body; I just needed closure really. By 9am my parents had arrived and mum brought along my older brother Justin. The nurses told me I wasn't allowed to eat, only drink water as I was going for surgery later that day. I was a little confused, so were my parents about the surgery. At 10am, the registrar came to explain that I would be having surgery to take a bit of bone marrow out to see if it has or has not spread to the bone. I would also be having a central line port inserted into my chest.

The central line port was something that completely threw me into the dark. I immediately hated it as she went on to explain what it does. It is a permanent line that is threaded through one of your main veins near your heart; it is used for giving chemotherapy and taking of blood. I will have it in temporarily till the end of treatment. I will also have two tubes sticking out my chest... I knew I was going to hate it, but I knew I'd have to have it.

I honestly wasn't as worried having the bone marrow surgery as I was more focused on what a central line was. She gave me a little pamphlet all about a central line port, and I'd have to say it was the ugliest thing I had ever seen! The front of the pamphlet showed a young sick boy who himself had one in his chest. Then the next two pages showed cartoons of it with detailing.

As I held myself together looking at the pamphlet, the registrar came in to explain that some results had come back. She explained they would organise for Dr Anazodo and the team to come and see me as soon as all results are received and will work this around the surgery. When she said this I was filled with excitement; Yes!!! Finally today I will have some answers!!

The day slowly dragged on, and I had this constant feeling of helplessness. I felt that there was no point in even crying or getting upset about this because there isn't much myself or my parents can do.

I can't go into my body and take the tumour out for good. I can't stop nor do anything to help the situation.

It was just before 1pm when I saw Dr Anazodo and her team walk in. They took me into another room that was situated down the end of the hall. It was a room full of lounges and chairs used for family meetings or for parents and carers who needed to stay overnight. We sat down in a big circle in the middle of the room, and I could sense the rise of anxiety and fear in the room.

Dr Anazodo didn't beat around the bush she got straight to the point. Immediately turning to me she said: "We have the full results of all the scans and tests done and have come to the final conclusion that you have Rhabdomyosarcoma Cancer."

My immediate reaction in my head was "well what the fuck is that?" I almost felt like bursting out laughing; who names a cancer that!? Like what is that! She continued to say that the tumour was slowly wrapping itself around the uterus, bladder and bowel. Because of this it was inoperable, and there was also a metastasis on the left fibula bone, and because of this I was Stage 4

By this stage, I felt numb and felt like a train had hit me full on. I didn't feel the need to cry or throw something across the room as I didn't feel it would get me anywhere. I didn't even feel sorry for myself; I wasn't sure how to feel in all honesty.

Ever since the moment of being told that my consciousness kept telling me "I'm going to be okay, you have to be okay; this isn't my life, I am not going to die this way." I have a PURPOSE. "I feel this feeling was the key." It was this that kept my drive to keep on fighting from the beginning. I knew I was going to be okay, the cancer isn't going to control me; I will control IT.

I say this in a very stern voice, as positive mindset is the key. I will always tell people that whether they have cancer or not if there is a will, there is a way.

No point in crying, no point in being negative about it because that will only fuel it and make the situation/cancer bigger.

Of course, there is a thing called "Doubt" but if you know and feel it, don't ever give up. Tell yourself you have many years ahead of you and push the doubt away; again it's all about the power of positive thinking.

As I slowly came back into the room to the conversation of Dr Anazodo I really couldn't remember the rest of the conversation as I had completely zoned out. Of course, I could hear what they were saying, but my mind had gone to different thoughts.

It felt like time had sped up. I remember her talking about the side effects of chemotherapy and also the possibility of changing hospitals and having treatment at John Hunter Newcastle. We lived nearly 2 hours away from Randwick so Dr Anazodo told us that John Hunter had exactly the same treatment and amazing team as they did and would be far easy to get too. I have to say she was exactly right.

My parents sat there in a daze and tried to write down as much as they could for fear of not remembering everything. As the conversation was coming to close one of the last things my mother asked was "How common is this disease and how many teens get it?" Dr Anazodo proceeded to say "It's very rare, we only estimate about nearly 20 people in Australia get it; mostly 2-10year old children"

It was then that my understanding of my cancer was lost. I am nearly 18 years old! Not 2, not 8 and not 10. I stumbled out of the room feeling quite sick and in a complete daze. I just needed to lie down. I awoke to see a wardsman at the end of the bed about to take me to surgery, pushing me out of the room with my dad walking behind. I remember my mum walking back in with a coffee, and started to cry; she just kept saying I was going to be okay over and over again.

She Will Always Carry On

As they wheeled me into the theatre, I began to stare into the bright lights above and as I did, a tall, middle-aged dark headed man walked out and introduced himself as the surgeon. He gave me a blue hair net to put on my head to tuck in my hair under it. He explained what a bone marrow is and what a port is. He asked me if I wanted to know how they put in a central line port in the chest... I immediately said no, thank you.

I remember dad holding me tightly as I said goodbye to him as they pushed me into the anaesthetic room.

Once in there a lovely lady nurse and anaesthetist both started talking to me, asking me many questions about what I do, finishing school, etc. Before I knew it everything started to become quite hazy and blurry and I started slurring my words; the lights grew darker and darker and then I was completely out to it.

I woke up immediately hearing my mum's voice next to me. I had this great huge throbbing feeling on the right side of my chest and a very stiff and sore bottom on the left side. I felt something hanging off my chest; it immediately freaked me out. I kept falling in and out of sleep. When I woke up again, and I was back in the ward and was a little more aware this time. I heard my mum's voice with the palm of her hand on my left cheek saying, "Maddy, we have to go home now and get your brother Justin home; the nurses said they think you will just sleep the rest of the evening anyway..." That was all I remember before I went back to sleep. I didn't wake up until 9am the next morning.

I woke up with immense pain in my chest, I could barely move it.

I also felt discomfort in the lower half of my back from where they took some bone marrow. I laid there feeling alone, trapped and vulnerable. I am living in a body that wants to destroy itself, and there is nothing I can do to stop it. The thought made me feel ill to the stomach and helpless.

My family walked in a short time later, the conversations we had, had nothing to do with cancer or being in the hospital. They were upbeat conversations about my formal (formal what?) in a few weeks time, my brother's work, etc..... It was like my family and I were almost pretending and trying to forget that I had a Stage IV cancer. Moments like this were the times I lived for, just forgetting for just a second about the reality I faced.

Later on that day my boyfriend at the time Mr X (not disclosing his name due to personal reasons) came to the hospital. I had already told him the news days before that I had a blue cell cancer tumour. He had a small idea of what my diagnosis would be as he was a full-time nurse working in a hospital.

By the time I was diagnosed, we had been together for roughly seven months, but it had been a rocky relationship from the start. My family didn't think he was right for me and thought there was too big an age gap. When he walked into my hospital room I was quite dazed because of all the painkillers I had been given; he gave me a big kiss and hug. It was just the two of us in the room when a baby-faced middle-aged man walked in. He proceeded to tell us that he is a gynaecologist and fertility doctor; I wasn't expecting him and was quite baffled by him too as he was male and I wasn't used to seeing a male gynaecologist. But hey, of course, I respect it and if they love it, then great! But I was a little intrigued.

He sat down and opened his folder to my profile and information. He then went on to explain what he does and how he can help with different options. I don't think anything prepared me for what he was about to tell me and those words will stay with me forever...

" Now Maddy, I have been looking at your diagnosis, the treatment plan, duration and what is to happen for you in the near future. Unfortunately, we have to rule out IVF as treatment has to start immediately and IVF takes up to 3 to 4 weeks to complete. Now there are a few other options available for you in the ways of protecting fertility and eggs.

But I need to tell you now Maddy, due to the severity, where your cancer is sitting, and due to it pushing up against your uterus, you have a very high chance of coming out of this completely childless. That in percentage form is roughly around 3%. And let's say if you go onto being that 3% and getting pregnant, the chances of miscarriage and stillborn are very high due to the pelvis area being completely destroyed and unable to hold the baby."

I immediately felt stripped of a huge part of me. I was numb, I didn't cry, I didn't scream. I just did what I did when I was diagnosed and that was to look at the blank wall across the room.

I guess having that ideal future of getting married, having kids, creating that amazing bond a woman and child has, breastfeeding and holding your own baby may be robbed from me. I can't tell you how stripped I felt and how robbed I felt; I never asked for this evil disease. This was more devastating than cancer itself. I could beat cancer but to never bear my own child was just too hard to bear.

My life will never be the same.

It took me a long time and days of crying to put this part into words; I am still today completely devastated and don't think I will ever get over it. I always wanted to have children in the future as I love kids, especially babies. Every person that I have told since that day and even just writing about it makes me cry.

On a spiritual and healing process I would imagine this beautiful spirit leaving my body to find someone else to wait their turn in this life. While I sit there and wave goodbye sadly hoping that those souls go onto a good life, a life without me. I think about this scenario a lot; for me, it's definitely on a spiritual and healing level and to also help myself cope and try to move on. It also helps give me hope that the very small chance could happen! Every time I think about this scenario I get a little stronger every time.

I do remember the Gynaecologist giving me some options but unfortunately there wasn't many, and most had a small success rate. I didn't have time to do IVF, but there was one option that stood out a little. It was a monthly injection into your lower back or butt that stops your period completely and reduces dramatically the blood flow to the area of your ovaries. It also minimises the risk of chemotherapy and radiation being drawn to the area and destroying the ovaries. This was the highest success rate of them all.

The gynaecologist gave me time to think about this and said he would come back tomorrow morning for my answer. I think I had already decided this would give me the best option of some hope.

That afternoon I got Mr X to tell my mum of the devastating news as I just couldn't talk about it to anyone at the time; it was too hard and especially telling your own mother that you may never have children. It was finally the day when I could get out of the hospital and just get home to my bed. The night before was awful, I cried all night. Never had I ever felt so alone and betrayed by my own body. I can't put into words the devastation and emotions that I felt that evening.

My dad, his partner Penny and my brother Justin got me that morning. We left at about 11:30am, and to be outside and smell the fresh air was simply phenomenal. On the way home we stopped at Mc Donald's, I remember thinking it would be the last time I would eat junk food as my doctors had recommended CLEAN EATING whilst having treatment. I have to admit it wasn't the last time as later down the track whilst on chemotherapy, I needed some junk food to put on weight...

Once home I fell into my bed and sunk right into my mattress and wow was that a beautiful moment. I burst into tears, and I cried so much that I made myself fall asleep because I was so sleep deprived. The next couple of days I loved being back at home and resting trying not to think of what was to come...

Chapter Two
Stolen Days

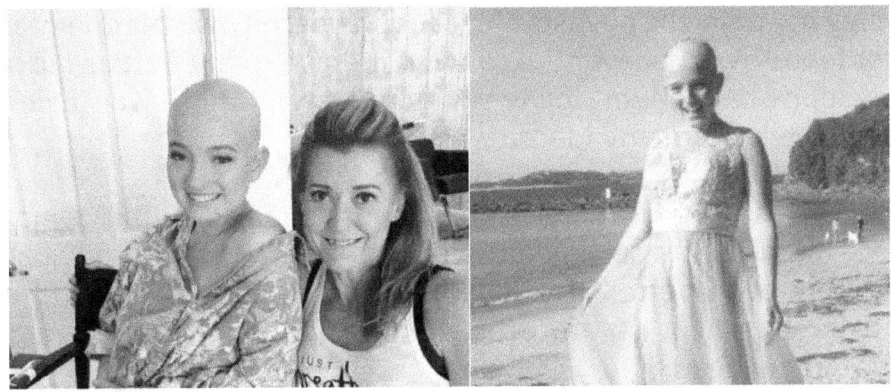

It was Sunday morning; I was awake for about an hour and had the whole time thinking of ways of how to break the news and diagnosis to my friends. I decided I would try to put in the lightest, yet most blunt way, through the use of Facebook and social media. I was never really sure about whether it was the right way to go about it, but I just figured everyone would eventually know and find out sooner or later. I planned to do it that evening in "peak" time so everybody would see and not missed out. I couldn't face going to each person individually; it was difficult enough telling my closest friends.

Mr X came over later that morning, and we decided to try spending some time together. My head kept telling me it might be the last days of feeling normal; who knew how I was going to feel after starting treatment.

That same morning I had also planned to cut off my long blonde hair. I wanted to do it myself and not let it fall out in clumps and thought just cutting in really short would be the best. I know it sounds kind of weird, but I wrapped my hair up in a plastic and put it away to keep... my hair at the time was my pride and joy, and it was a part of me and the person I was then. Cutting it off was a good decision and doing it early stopped me feeling too much emotional pain. Anyway, it needed a real good chop as I had an African lady braid it tightly months(i think something is not really okay with "it tightly months") before and it had caused dryness and splitting.

Losing my hair was devastating as I considered my hair one of my best features. I had wanted to grow it down to my butt as I loved long hippy hair!! Mum slowly cut it off, and I felt like I was losing a part of myself and my identity.

After staring at myself for a solid hour, I started to find a small piece of acceptance. I kept telling myself it will grow back, probably even better after chemotherapy (so they say) and it's only temporary; it isn't forever... I think I said it to myself over 50 times in my head.

I want to share with anybody in the world who may be facing the same fears and encourage them to embrace it. I started to feel empowered and more feminine than ever before being bald, don't abide by societies stereotypes and expectations. Even under such horrible circumstances embrace this certain side effect! It will only happen for a small period of time and remember it WILL grow back... it's also very convenient to no more shaving underarms or legs, waxing eyebrows, bikini waxing ;)

" I forgave my body, I forgave it for trying to destroy itself. I thanked it as without it I'm not the person I am today."

- Maddy Ritchie

Mr X showed up just after my hair ordeal. He was a man who at times was filled with much kind and loving words, yet he was a person that you felt you weren't sure if he ever meant what he said... says a lot about our relationship at the time huh!

We decided to go to a local waterfall in Somersby about a 20-minute drive from where I live. We had a nice picnic and I immersed myself in fresh water and the beautiful air but constantly thinking this bloody tube hanging out of my chest is driving me nuts and was also very sore.

I stood under the falls as the freshwater come over my head and body, and I held my arms out and wept. I closed my eyes, and all I could hear was the splashing of water and the birds singing in the trees.

In these moments I felt like fear had completely left me and the fear of the unknown was being washed away, and I began to pray. Before my diagnosis, I was an atheist and didn't have much faith, but on that day my spirituality completely changed, it was like a spiritual awakening. As I prayed I felt a strong sense of healing over my body and something I just cannot explain or put into words. It felt like a light bulb moment for me, a feeling I'm not alone, and I am going to be okay and to never stop believing. As I came out of the waterfall, I felt at peace. It was only just the beginning of my spiritual journey and more wonderful whacky things were yet to come.

When I arrived home, I was very tired and felt weak. Some relatives and friends were visiting as my mum had already told some people of the news. As I came out of my room later that afternoon I sat outside around the table with them all; a few were asking how I felt or if there was anything they could do. This was my first experience with others looking at me with such despair and sadness. It honestly annoyed me a lot... like yes I have a horrible disease, and I was unlucky but don't feel sorry for me as I am not going to be just fine, let's talk about something other than cancer the whole time you're here.

I would later learn to accept that that is a natural human way of dealing with this horrible disease and the shock of someone so young getting cancer. I learnt to not get upset or annoyed it's just a normal human response.

It was the worst day of the week... MONDAY. Justin, Mum, Anthony, my dad, and myself all got up early that morning and made the trip up to John Hunter Hospital, Newcastle about an hour and half drive from my place.

We had no idea what to expect, but we only knew that I'd be admitted to start my first chemo treatment. We were all on edge on the way up in the car.

Once there, we met with Dr Frank Alvaro the Head of Paediatric Oncology who had been in contact with Dr Antoinette Anazodo's team at Randwick Children's Hospital Sydney. He was a lovely and welcoming man, a warm personality and had these big wide glasses on.

We all huddled into a small interview room in the day unit, eagerly awaiting his comments. He bought up my scans on the computer screen and looked very intent on them zooming in and out and looking at notes. He turned straight to me and said "Maddy, you will be admitted today of course and starting your first chemotherapy treatment this afternoon. I know that Dr Anazodo gave you a big briefing on chemotherapy and its side effects etc..." as his voice began to lower and crack a little as he went on to say "If this treatment protocol we are about to begin Maddy, does not work or the cancer continues to grow I give you no more than three months to live due to the severity of the size and the type of cancer you have. You have a success rate of making it past three months of only 5%..."

I instantly didn't believe him, I stared straight back at him with utter confusion and disbelief. I was not fully aware of the severity of my survival rate. I just stared vigorously back at him. I still struggle even now with the low percentage of my survival rate, but I am determined that I am going to be that 5%.

Mum was stunned, and I heard her say "WHAT"!?   I remember looking around the room and back at Frank thinking you've got the wrong patient, my survival rate can't be that low.

Once the meeting was over, I just tried to pretend it didn't happen that the conversation ceased to exist. My mindset was that if it's my time to go, then I'll go but at least I died trying...

it was just a way for me to comfort myself or to have some sort of justification within myself if I did die within the next 3 months I certainly gave it my all.

Dr Alvaro's Clinical Nurse Carly showed us around the hospital and the ward I would be staying in overnight. I would have my own room which made me pretty ecstatic when compared to when I had to share a room with five other kids at Randwick. Here, there was even a bed so mum could stay with me overnight.

It was around 4:30pm that afternoon when the nurses walked in in their protective outfit to put up my first chemotherapy. At first, I found their outfits a little intimidating as I felt like I had a spreadable disease or swine flu, but I soon learnt that they wore these outfits to protect themselves from severe burns should the chemo leak from the packaging onto their skin.

I couldn't help noticing my mum taking photos from all angles. God love her....I knew these photos would become a huge part of my journey and give me memories and achievements to look back on.

The first few hours I didn't really feel too much but then I suddenly started to take a turn for the worst. It wasn't so much immediate vomiting for me, it was slowly fatigue, nausea, and tiredness and then the thought of food making my whole body feel ill. Everything kind of slowed down a little and I tended to feel like a zombie.

The next morning I felt even more deathlike, and looking in the mirror I looked like a ghost. My mum wasn't coming into the hospital until the afternoon. I noticed time was definitely not on my side, it seemed to drag and go really slowly. Being by myself made it worse and didn't help my mental health. I kept thinking of what my friends would be doing and how they'd be having fun either travelling or partying, and I was sitting in this hospital room feeling like rubbish. It seemed so unfair.

Whilst on the ward different people would come in to try and help take your mind off things, and one of those days I was given a notepad, pens and beautiful colouring in books (from the amazing Starlight Foundation). I was still having trouble accepting my cancer and couldn't understand why me,m so I got the notepad and immediately began to write out my feelings of pain and emotions, and it helped me cope and feel a little at ease.

My first entry reads:

20th October 2015 11:03am

Understanding the cancer I have been diagnosed with is just too hard for me to fathom... I have no genetic line on either side of my family nor have I done anything to cause this Stage 4 Rhabdomyosarcoma Cancer.

There is recent evidence suggesting the biology and cells dividing within the muscle tissues as you grow cause it although there is little evidence to support that...

Around 23 people in Australia get Rhabdomyosarcoma mostly aged between 2 and 12 years old. What the fuck did the 23 of us do to get this!?? I have a 5% chance of making it to February of 2016 and have a survival life span of up to 5 years from diagnosis due to the high prognosis of relapse. I really truly feel that I have been given this for a PURPOSE.

I will control this cancer; it is not going to control neither my life nor myself. I am also a big believer of the mind and that the mind holds the key to success or failure. Love and cherish the life you have and what you have been given. The amount of love and support I got from posting on my Facebook about my diagnosis was beyond overwhelming and amazing. Thank you.

Once out of the hospital the next day, FINALLY! Mr X took me out for dinner that evening. I had a sudden and random craving for a big juicy steak, it was only the beginning of my weird and whacky cravings from chemotherapy. We went to the local pub, and after ordering and sitting down, I had an overwhelming feeling of just wanting to cry and breakdown. Mr X kind of just sat there with little empathy on his face and of course I didn't expect him to understand, I didn't expect anybody to understand, it was my grief and pain and that's more than okay.

I don't know why he lacked empathy; he was always a little vague anyway and away with the fairies (so to speak). He went on to say "well Maddy it will be over in January, don't worry you will be right". I felt like cancer to him wasn't a big deal. I was also gobsmacked when he went on to say we should have kids at the end of my treatment... ummm have you lost the plot? I will be 19 and recovering from cancer in the PELVIS; kids would be the last thing on my mind and in all honesty, I knew in myself that we wouldn't be together at the end of my treatment.

I do regret not breaking up with him then and there. Our personalities and goals were just way to far apart and who in their right mind says that to someone? Oh and I forgot to mention he was a lot older than me too...

In his teen years, he used to tell me he got into a lot of heavy drugs, I always felt that affected who he was today, his emotions, understanding of others, his goals and also how he dealt with situations and hard times.

As I sat there balling in the middle of the pub I just ended up walking off to the women's bathrooms to pull myself together. As I came back the food arrived; I barely ate any of it anyway and from that day forward I never could finish a full meal.

I had a hard time the days following my first chemotherapy treatment. I barely moved from my bed and felt very fatigued, and every time I stood up, I almost felt like I was going to collapse and pass out.

After each chemotherapy, I had to have an injection called Neulasta into the top of my thigh. It helps bring your white cell count back up and helps your body recover quicker. It's also used to help you have a good count for your next chemotherapy to go ahead. We would go home after treatment and put on numbing cream to the area, and mum would have to do the injection. She became a nurse overnight, but I know she hated doing it as she didn't want to hurt me.

Every time I have Neulasta it makes my bones ache really badly, and my bones become really weak, even holding a cup of water in my hand hurt.

The beginning of treatment was very tough to say the least, as each week of chemotherapy treatment rolls around, you go into this vicious cycle of never ending feeling like crap then becoming okay again just to feel like crap again.

The weeks went by quickly, particularly as you don't have a routine and seem to live each day by going to the hospital. After every treatment, I was also afraid that I would become sick and be back in the hospital again. I know the nurses and doctors do a great job, but I hated being in the hospital and would always become very emotional. I tried to live each day as it came but in those early months, I was scared the treatment wouldn't work, and my cancer would continue growing.

The whole situation hit me like a fast train (I look back now and think about those moments and cry for myself and the helplessness that I felt).

My hair was completely gone; I felt unattractive at times, was living with a relationship that was on the rocks, afraid of the future and feeling sometimes that I just wanted to die. I had 100% complete support from my friends and family, but my mentality and will to live would tend to fade in and out at times. I prayed a lot, I prayed for healing, and I prayed to find a reason.

Going out the shops those first few times to say the least was very interesting and yes a lot of people did look at me with pity or sadness. I guess I could say I am in general quite a confident person and didn't care too much about what others thought. I cared more about myself and how I thought and felt. Even in those days of feeling down and having barely any self-esteem I still kept walking out bald; it gave me strength.

I always felt I didn't want to hide my reality behind an itchy wig and it was through those first few times that I developed an understanding that it is human nature to feel empathy. At first, I did get very upset and angry with people who did pity me, I just wanted to be normal but at the end of the day, I'm not, I am unwell, and that is ok.

I always tell others in similar situations as me or who want to be bald but are afraid of society's stereotypes to just do it! You only live once, don't let other people's thoughts and opinions towards you have that power over you. Only you have that choice, show them who is boss! I cannot say enough!!

It's Sunday and tomorrow I have 6 days of chemotherapy...

My 18th birthday was on the Sunday and formal the day after. If anything I had my birthday to look forward to and tried to focus on that, but nothing could prepare me for those brutal 6 days ahead of me.

On the way to the hospital on Monday morning I experienced pre-hospital sickness. I was so afraid of going into hospital that I became nauseous, I hate hospital... A LOT.

I was to have chemotherapy Monday-Friday and then a 24hr fluid flush until Saturday morning. Each day was slow and was a downhill spiral of getting sicker and sicker. I felt alone; it was a bleak and depressing environment. I had my mum there at times, but even for her it got a bit hard. I felt trapped in these four walls, I wasn't even allowed to leave to go outside. The days were pointless, and it was the same bullshit over and over again.

I tried to keep myself busy and entertained by listening to music or watching a TV series, but even after a while, you do get bored of that. Anything I did to help tackle against the boring and mental pain was a struggle. At times it was probably one of the lowest points in my life; I always held onto the fact that there were better days ahead and it will get better, it's only temporary. Without this mindset and thought in the back of my mind, I honestly don't think I would get through this treatment.

I truly believe that no matter what situation you are in, no matter what religion or situation you may be facing, always believe in yourself and find meaning even in the small things. When you don't have any purpose or meaning, it can take you into deep water, and it can destroy you at times. It nearly did for me, don't let the evilness of the world and people overtake your faith and mindset, don't ever let it hurt you. Remain strong.

Saturday finally came, and I felt a huge feeling of accomplishment after finishing that big week of chemotherapy. I was also beyond excited for the next couple of days.

Mr X came and picked me up from the hospital, and I busted out at about midday. As I walked out of the hospital, my whole body was just filled with amazement. The fresh air and the glaring sun was honestly the most magnificent feeling for me, just walking outside again was something I was beyond thankful for.

My eyes became sore as it was struggling to get used to the glare. When I got out, I was craving pizza like crazy, a big juicy meat lovers and Hawaiian... YES PLEASE.

We got pizzas and ended up having a little picnic at this beautiful reserve about 5km down the road from the hospital. The place was filled with many families and children having birthdays surrounded by nature. It was so surreal, coming out of hospital and into the outside world and nature became so much more beautiful to me.

The fresh air and the beauty of nature and just the country that I am so fortunate to live in is amazing. I took it all for granted before all of this happened to me. Just being outside gives you a real sense of healing and peace; just being around nature. That's another thing I struggle to understand that we humans are destroying the earth... for greed! As I close my eyes and lay down on the grass, I fall away to the sounds of nature and kids playing in the distance.

Today is my eighteenth birthday, and I wake up feeling like hell on earth. My bones ache, I felt nauseous and very weak. I pushed myself to just get up out of bed; honestly, I could have stayed in bed and completely forgotten that it even was my birthday. As I stood up to get changed, I looked in my wardrobe and felt a drop in my blood pressure and immediately sat back down. Something that would normally take me between 10 minutes to get changed took me 30 minutes; I started to become very frustrated with myself.

It was around midday when my close family and friends arrived. Some hadn't seen me in a while, and I distinctly remember my aunty breaking down in tears when she saw me. I guess it was hard for her and my family to see the beginning of changes in me.

It was an emotional day and very overwhelming. It was the first time I ever broke down in front of my family since the diagnosis until then I had my emotions completely hidden; I am good at it too. I got beautiful presents and cards from everyone. It was a day filled with much love but also a day of loss for me.

I am not allowed to drink alcohol while on treatment; I have to be honest it would have been awesome to celebrate with a drink. The whole day I felt weak and not very excited about my birthday at all. I felt a little robbed actually, I mean it's my 18th birthday and should have been a big deal. A memory that was supposed to be good and fun felt stolen from me.

That evening Mr X took me out for pizza and to the local beer garden to play the pokies. By this stage, I could have collapsed in a heap, but I kept going and pushed myself as I wanted to do something to celebrate my 18th. On the way from the car to the beer garden a friend of Mr X came up to us, I remember meeting him a few months back, he was a lovely guy. When he saw me, I don't think I have ever seen someone's face go from smiling to utter and complete devastation.

He was a grown man in his early 20s, and he broke down and cried in the middle of the busy walkway. He kept grabbing my hand and saying that he didn't understand the world and why me and I am such a good person! This young man made me realise how devastating and hard it is for everyone around me to watch me go through this journey. I felt sad for myself; I didn't want to make others sad because of my situation...

The beer garden had Sunday sessions on; it's like a weekly ritual on the coast for all the young people to go to around the Terrigal and Central Coast area. When we walked in I never felt so confronted with this feeling of intimidation and judgemental looks especially from other girls around my age.

The ones that did look at me were kind of all dressed the same and seemed like they followed in packs and lived for every Sunday night to get drunk. I just tried to ignore them the best I could.

I was wearing tracksuit pants and well wasn't looking my best that night.... I honestly didn't care! We hurried through to the gaming room, once in there I had a $10 but I had no idea what to do. Mr X gave me a brief explanation but really all I did was press random buttons. Before I know it, the machine started to make all these crazy noises then the screen was going from $50-$150 and up and up! It then got to $300 and by this time I wasn't even pressing anything.

I could not believe it I walked away with $300 and truly believe that everything happens for a reason; I went on to find out why the next day.

It was formal day, and I'd never got around to getting a formal dress due to obvious reasons. I did have this white lace dress in my cupboard that I was thinking about wearing but it was quite revealing and not exactly the formal type.

Mum thought with the money I got from the pokies last night we should go out and find a dress. There weren't many formal dress shops on the coast, and we didn't want to drive to Sydney or Newcastle.

I was searching away on my phone for any shops that did formal wear. After making a few phone calls we finally got onto one that did have bridal and formal wear and was about a 25minute drive from where we were.

We arrived; it was called Ferrari Formal wear in Somersby Industrial Park.

The ladies in there were beautiful and so lovely to us. My mum really wanted me to try on baby pink formal dresses but I was more lenient towards red. After trying on many dresses, the lady brought over two new in season baby pink formal dresses. The first one was stunning, but I couldn't fit nor zip up around my bust area. But the second one I immediately loved, it was beautiful material, elegant and it also covered my centraline!

The dress was definitely not in our price range, it was $600 and we only had at the most $350. The ladies had a secret chat and really wanted me to have this dress so they gave it us for a cost price of $300. The dress needed to be taken up at the bottom, so they even did that for me at no cost. The ladies were absolutely amazing and beautiful, I don't know what I would have done or worn to the formal if it wasn't for them both...

Because we waited for the dress to be taken up, we were starting to run out of time. We stopped off quickly at a nail parlour on the way home to fix up my ridiculously long nails and then went straight home. It was a crazy hot day and the heat made me feel worse.

I already had shoes, thank God! And they went perfectly with the dress. As I attempted to put on makeup, my eyelashes began to fall out, and I struggled to feel pretty. The vision I had for what I'd look like at my formal 6 months ago was definitely not the same now.

I was already tired, and it was only 4:30pm and I was concerned about wearing my long formal dress in the heat.

We went to Terrigal Haven first for photos with everyone from my year. When I got out of the car, the heat hit me like a ton of bricks. My dress felt like it was sticking to my skin from the heat. I walked steadily over but scared I was going to fall on my heels in front of everyone.

I had not seen most of them since graduation and I noticed some of them were a little afraid of coming near me as I don't think they knew what to say or do; I expected that, and it was ok.

When some of the girls came up to me, it became a crying fest; although we were all trying so hard not to ruin our makeup.

After taking an awful lot of photos, we all made our way to the Crowne Plaza where the formal itself would be held. Most of us drove that few seconds down the road instead of walking and by the time we arrived, I'd become quite fatigued from the heat; it almost felt like I had sun stroke.

We all made our way upstairs to the function room and sat at our assigned tables. I was sitting with a few of my friends which was great. While we listened to the principal congratulating us all, I couldn't help but notice the boys across from me on another table with flasks of whiskey in their suits trying secretly to drink from them. Needless to say, they were caught and told to leave.

Towards the end of the main presentation, two girls stood up and announced the awards that were voted by us. Some were pretty ridiculous, and I wasn't sure whether some people just voted for themselves. As they got to the last award they asked everyone to stand up; with much confusion we all did. The two girls went on to say "we present this to a girl who has been given something so horrific, yet has stayed so strong; we present the award for beauty and bravery to Maddy Ritchie".

For about a split second I was a little confused I definitely didn't think it would be me. As I about to match forward, I immediately broke down and cried as I had absolutely no idea this was going to happen.

As I stumble towards the 200 kids standing and screaming behind me, it was really an amazing feeling. I never liked school at all, and I felt like honestly nobody cared at all about me.

This was a moment I will never forget; I definitely felt like everybody did care.

As I cry into the microphone and say "thank you" everyone started screaming again and then someone took a photo and I thought

"Oh whoa! That's going to look so dashing, me and my crying face... hahaha"

At the after party, most people were smashed or on the verge of becoming very drunk. Personally, it sucked for me just sitting there with my lime and soda water, I'm not a big drinker anyway, but in times like these it's always fun to let your hair down. I didn't really like the after party, I felt like I couldn't join in on the fun like I should be doing, I just wanted to have fun with my friends.

I was on a week break, and mum decided to take me to the beach with our new umbrella as it was crazy hot. It was my first time being back at the beach since before diagnosis. The beach is an amazing place, a good sense of healing and fresh air. Due to having a central line in my chest I'm not allowed to swim owing to the high risk of infection and can only go in water just below my chest.

I sat on the shore that day and cried as I loved the beach, and I loved swimming especially when there were waves. I don't think people realise that being able to swim openly in a beautiful beach is such a gift. People take the beach for granted; I did before my diagnosis, and now all I wanted was to swim under the waves and immerse myself in the water; honestly it's very hard.

My chemo cycle was three days one week, one day the next week and 6 days the following week, all in a four-week period.

Each time I received the same chemotherapy drugs, my body became more used to it, and I found that my side effects settled a bit after the second time around, but it was still awful.

The second day I was in for my three-day chemo. I struggled with my feelings especially when I saw on Facebook and Snap Chat how all my friends were organising their end of school trips to Bali or somewhere overseas. It was something that I should have been doing too not sitting in a hospital bed having chemo drugs put into my body. I should have been out there living as an 18-year-old; I tried so hard to ignore my feelings, but It really did upset me. I cried a lot about this, but I know soon that one day I will be doing that, I will be living again.

I had been following this health and living page on Facebook called "Health Science" it was very insightful and shared quite a fair bit on ways to help cure cancer naturally with backed up research. One day these two articles appeared on my news feed, one was about the power of frankincense oil and the other being all about this oil called black cumin seed. I researched them both and found some good evidence to back up what they were saying. Both suggested that it helped in destroying cancer cells and tumours and frankincense can also help with nausea and fatigue. Mum and I went to the local organic store to buy them, and I made sure both were authentic and pure with no added ingredients.

Once I got my hands on them, I rushed home and began to use them in the hope they were both going to help me in my cancer fight.

I applied frankincense to the pelvic area and put four drops over the residing tumour. I rubbed it in softly and held my hand for about 30 seconds over the area and did some deep breathing. I also took a spoonful of black cumin seed with honey every day; it was awful and made me gag sometimes, but honey with it helped me to swallow it.

I had a lot of faith in both of these practises, and I did it every day, I also believe that cancer is caused by nature and to help undo that or destroy it why not use something natural to do that?

90% of the time I barely moved from my bed after chemotherapy each week, my days were filled with watching documentaries, VICE or The Walking Dead. Someday I couldn't even do that, as I couldn't bear to look at the screen as my eyes became sensitive to unnatural light. I never really vomited as much as I thought I would after chemotherapy, which was a little odd as I did expect that to happen more but obviously my body reacted differently. I did struggle with my blood pressure as it dropped a lot just moving in and out of bed and especially when I had shower. Some days I didn't have a shower as I was too weak or afraid I would collapse.

The meaningful days of recovering and healing from the last bout of chemotherapy only to be torn down again by the next one takes a toll on your mental health. I cried every time as I had to go to hospital, I really did not like it all I also had a fear of it too.

I learnt from diagnosis who my real friends were and who wasn't. I got closer to some and others completely disappeared from my life. My boyfriend at the time MR X is one on the other hand, I can't put into words. From diagnosis, our relationship went completely downhill over the first few months. I truly didn't think we were together anyway for most of it, he was mainly just a friend to me. I just don't think he could handle the situation although he never admitted. Yes, there were good times, but most of it could never make up for majority of the bad.

He disrespected me on a whole other level in my first few months of diagnosis. Chemotherapy definitely affects your intimacy. My monthly needle to turn everything off leaves you menopausal with no desire or drive to even think about sex.

I do believe that intimacy is a big part of a relationship, but with my situation, it was something I couldn't help or change. There were times where Mr X failed to understand that or support me. At times I would cry as he would make me feel bad about the situation.

I should have left him and rid him completely from my life that day, but I was afraid; afraid of being lonely and by myself, afraid nobody else would want to be with me. Never will I ever let a man make me feel the way he did. I will never let a person take my worth and dignity from me ever again. I am stronger than ever now because of you; I regret deeply staying with him for as long as I did. It was the one thing I failed from the start to do, rid my life of the toxic people. I would tell anybody now to let him or her go! Whether it be a boyfriend/girlfriend, friend, acquaintance, family member or whoever in your life is causing you long term pain, is not changing and is hurting you or others around you, get rid of them.

Fill yourself and your life with POSITIVE people. I learnt that the hard way of how devastating it is if you don't. Don't keep holding out for somebody to change. Life's too short.

The week leading up to scans was a scary and very fearful time; these results were going to determine the course in which my life will go from here on. I felt good, and I truly believed that these scans were going to be good. I felt it in my body, and the lump had reduced in size and wasn't pushing out from my pelvis. I had been doing my frankincense oil, black cumin seed, prayer, meditation and alkaline water.

My mum was very on edge about the scan results too. I knew it would be very hard for my mum, as she gave birth to me, watched me grow and to see her own daughter be in pain and possibly die must have made her feel very helpless. I always reassured her that it would work out fine and good days were ahead; I do worry about my mum a lot.

Scan day arrived! I woke up almost feeling excited in a weird way, I really tried to keep positive, and I knew it would be a good outcome, I could just feel it!!

Justin, Mum, Anthony and myself drove up that morning and met up with my father and his partner Penny.

We all waited patiently and silently in the waiting room eager to know; Mum especially looked very anxious and worried.

Dr Frank walked around the corner and appeared bright and cheerful, which was kind of a good sign.

We all quickly huddled into the small oncology room fit for four people and sat in silence as we waited for Dr Frank to talk. After attempting multiple times to get the scans up on the computer Dr Frank finally got it open. He bought up my very first scan at diagnosis and then the scan I just had and compared the two. His face looked a little shocked at the comparisons. I just stared at him glaring, avoiding the screen. He began to nod his head up and down with a straight grin on his face, he turned to me, and he said in a very startled manner,

"The tumour had shrunk, most of it has actually disappeared Maddy"

A huge smile immediately came across my face, I felt like singing "alleluia, alleluia, alleluia" ha-ha, what an amazing relief and accomplishment.

Dr Frank turned the computer towards me and pointed out the comparison in the two scans from diagnosis to now and it was quite an amazing difference. He pointed out that he could still see a little pea-size tumour in what remained, but nothing like the original tennis ball sized tumour. Mum began to cry, and everyone in the room just had these wonderful smiles on their faces.
It honestly felt like a God was watching over me, such a big result in such little time was beyond amazing. BYE RHABDOMYOSARCOMA.

Dr Frank went on to explain that I would still need to continue with the same protocol and chemotherapy regime until the beginning of February and then he would start looking at a date for radiation treatment.

Hearing that, I had to continue to do the same regime. Even after this scan came back so positive, it was a little bit of a letdown for me as I really wanted it to all be over. I told myself at least now I know I am heading in the right direction and not living each day not knowing whether I will be here tomorrow; I still have a long road ahead, but I will get better.

Chapter Three

Life Before

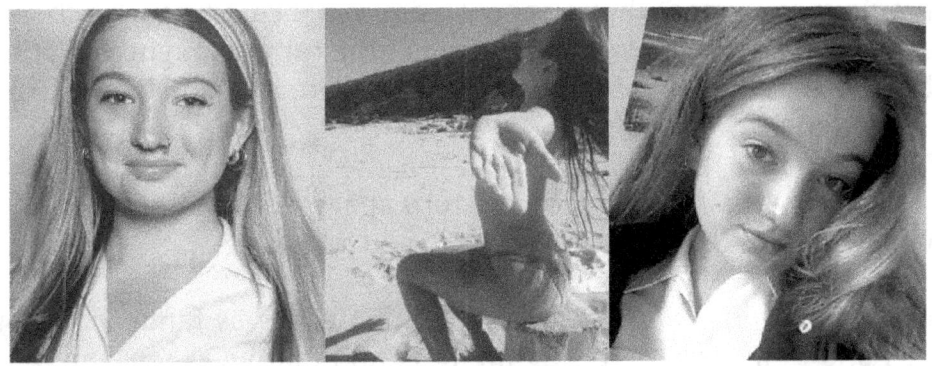

My life before cancer and all the memories I have of it felt like a long time ago to me now.

My high school life before cancer was very up and down. I had been at my local school Terrigal High for my final year of schooling and out of all the schools I went to, it was probably the best.

I had always struggled with fitting in and I was always the girl who was left out of a lot of things. Once I got to year 11, I came to breaking point and had a sudden realisation of just not caring anymore.

I don't know what the sudden realisation was, but I guess I just woke up one day and decided to care about what I think of myself more than anybody else. I was a vivacious and very outgoing person, and I did know that I was also very carefree too which a lot of people didn't like.

I was the girl that sang 'My Sharona' or 'The Pina Colada Song'...

I asked a lot of questions in class and questioned teachers a lot.

I do look back on those days and feel I pushed the boundaries a lot especially with some of the questions I asked. I laugh to myself now about who I was and how I've changed. At the time I guess that's all I knew, I didn't want to conform, I didn't want to follow the crowd, I wanted to break the rules and be myself.

Previous to Terrigal High School I went to a local Christian school. Why I did, I don't know but my mum at the time 'thought' it would be a better education for me not that we were religiously Christian at the time.

In the end, this school made me turn against Christianity and the whole idea of religion altogether.

Most people there were stuck in a bubble, it was fantasyland of lies and being protected by mummy and daddy. When I arrived at the school, having come from a performing arts school, which was the previous school I went to, some were very cautious of me. I will never forget this one occasion which happened in my first week of being in the school as a girl in my grade said to another girl right in front of my face " don't talk to her, let's go, she's not religious" they then both walked off.

I did go on to meeting some really beautiful people though who were religious and had the loveliest souls I had ever met.

The experience I took away from being at this school wasn't a nice one. My uniform never seemed to be correct, always feeling like you have to be this certain person and do things a certain way and even when studying religion it was a very one-sided class talk and never easy to have an opinion. If I voiced my opinion, I could even end up with a detention or feeling that a teacher didn't like me personally. From this experience I did turn atheist and lost a lot of faith; that was when I moved onto Terrigal High to be my own person and have a voice.

I went on to meet my first boyfriend in my final year of school, he was a lovely boy, and we really had some awesome times together. We only lasted about 7months and both went our separate ways as we both felt it wasn't right and were two different people by the end. After that relationship had ended, a couple of months later, I went on to meet Mr X. It was full steam ahead and very fast at the beginning.

She Will Always Carry On

I was a little naive at the time when we got together and was still a little sad by how the previous relationship ended.

I never cared too much about my grades at school, I just wanted to get through my final year. I skipped quite a lot of classes or signed out early and went home. I was losing interest and becoming sick and tired of school life; that was the time my cancer began to grow.

In the final months of school, I noticed I began to fall apart physically and at the time I did not understand why. I drifted from a lot of my friends and at recess and lunch went to the library.

It was at times very embarrassing, but I was tired of all the schoolyard talk and preferred the solitude of the library.

I struggled spiritually to understand who I was and the meaning of my life at this time. I struggled with a sense of purpose.

I was always a very grounded and chilled person, but my feelings deep down would creep in, and I felt very confused.

I held on to a lot of my past traumas and heartache. I may seem altogether on the outside but on the inside I felt very hollow and lonely and struggled to fill and understand the missing pieces in my life.

I had some good friends, but I always knew that when school was over, they would disappear from my life completely. I never really had a full connection with majority of my friends anyway, and as people, our interests and what we wanted in life was never quite the same.

I always tried to enjoy who I was, my attitude about life; I think that was what truly kept me grounded and kept me going.

Always know that if you ever find yourself in a stage in your life where you feel alone, believe me you're not! When it comes to high school, they're other girls and boys silently out there feeling the same as you, facing similar things and situations.

I wanted to break up with Mr X so many times in that final year of high school. My friends didn't particularly like him, and they all thought he was little crazy. They all worried about me being with him.

I often think how at the beginning of the relationship that wonderful person that drew me towards him wasn't who he truly was.

We took at least five different breaks over a span of about four months and the relationship between us became very toxic and unhealthy.

He was somebody that was very emotional, good with his words, overreacted a lot and was quite feminine at times. I think being the feminine man he was, caused things to spiral even more.

I started to question his sexuality as I found some things and heard stories that began to confirm this for me. It freaked the hell out of me at times and again I thought I should end the relationship once and for all. The main reason I didn't was loneliness and a fear of being on my own. I felt like nobody else would want to love me or even go out with me as I was the girl with cancer.

If I could turn back time, I would have made myself think differently, staying with someone when you both clearly know it's toxic and just not working just for the sake of it or to feel that void within yourselves is the worst thing you could ever do. You are better off without them, don't ever let anybody sweet-talk or gift their way back into your life either!!

I had also decided to get a tattoo around this time... Why? Because why not! I had always wanted one for a long time, and it means something to me on a personal level. I'm also a big fan of tattoos as they can have such beauty and art! A friend at school gave me the contact details for this tattoo artist that worked from home, he did do one for her, and he's very good. He also doesn't care too much about age (wink wink). I chose a sunflower, and we both sat there and looked at the drawings of them and he showed me sketches of some he had done. We eventually found one that I wanted, and I never looked back!

I got an orange sized sunflower on the top of my left thigh, it was one of the most uncomfortable two hours of my life; it hurt!

The sunflower represents life, light, and earth.

Did I forget to mention I didn't tell my mum until three months after?

I was one of only three of two hundred kids in my grade that had a tattoo, and I felt empowered by it and it gave me confidence within myself.

As I look back now, there were certain warning signs that something wasn't quite right in my body. I was constantly feeling run down and very tired. Whenever I returned home from half a day at school, I usually take a nap especially if I was going out that night.

At the time I didn't think it was a big deal. I just put it down to my lifestyle and everything happening at school with final exams, graduation, parties, relationships and personal stuff. I just thought I was really stressed out and had a lot happening at that time.

At the end of August, I went in for a tonsillectomy. Over the years I was often sick of tonsillitis and because of so many bouts the back of my tonsils had become infected.

I needed a tonsillectomy to remove it all.

The tonsillectomy didn't go as planned, about a week after the operation I was back in hospital, due to a massive bleed and blood clot where the tonsils were removed. It's not a rare thing; you can have a bleed after a tonsillectomy, but it's not a good thing either.

To this day I believe having this setback didn't help with my cancer, I'm not saying it caused my cancer but something in my body changed from this procedure.

I rapidly declined physically by the beginning of September and noticed I'd gained a lot of weight, and my stomach seemed abnormally bloated. I honestly thought I looked pregnant, but I knew I wasn't as we had taken precautions.

I started to feel useless, and very short of breath; even walking upstairs at school seemed a challenge which definitely should not have been for someone of my age.

At the time I always had a good relationship with my mum. I told her everything, and we got along really well. There were definitely ups and downs, but that's a normal thing with a teenage daughter; we were always pretty solid.

After my parents broke up, I barely saw my dad. He worked in the Navy and was constantly away. We didn't always have the most stable relationship anyway especially in my early teens. Due to the personal reasons of why my parents broke up made me hold a lot of anger towards what my father did at the time. I definitely struggled at the beginning with forgiving him and hurting my mum and I felt like this for quite a few years. It took my cancer diagnosis for us both to start rebuilding and regaining that relationship back.

It was graduation day, and was I excited to leave this hell place and get out in the world and do amazing things.

I wanted to be with people I wanted to be with, and learn amazing things that will help me through life. I never wanted to go to University or do hundreds of essays or re-read Shakespeare's plays that you have read or heard for the 20th time. I wanted to experience the world.

I was undoubtedly proud of myself for making it to that final day as 2 years prior I just wanted to give up. It also helped me to move forward and move past what I went through throughout my schooling years and leave it all behind for new beginnings.

At the time I had no idea what I wanted career wise. Everybody seemed to have it all together and got into the university they wanted and had a plan, but I didn't. The main thing I wanted to do was look at travelling and volunteering overseas. I had already applied to go to Spain and work in a youth hostel and do volunteer work for my accommodation; I just needed to save for a plane ticket.

At the graduation ceremony, some of the girls in my grade were crying while I just sat there with a huge grin on my face thinking get me out of here already!!

At my school and the local schools around the area, after graduation, the whole grade joins in with what we call "Fridge to Fridge". We all ride around on bikes going to about five different stops where you drink, dance and have fun with everybody. It would have been one of the most ridiculous days of my life. Being very stupid I decided to down all my drinks in one go. I stumbled with everybody else from one stop to another, almost being hit by cars or forgetting how to ride my bike, could have been very dangerous; it would have been a pretty ridiculous sight for the sober civilians around at the time.

I have no recollection of most of it as I was completely smashed. I don't even remember the last stop.

This was all two weeks prior to my diagnosis, and it's honestly a wonder I didn't pass out or end up in the hospital; I had severely pushed my body to its limit.

I was always quite comfortable in my own skin, but I wasn't always like that. Throughout Year 9 to Year 11 I was a mess within myself as I struggled with anxiety and body issues. I never really shared it too much with anybody or showed my weakness, I was very good at hiding it.

I was outspoken and was at one stage very passionate about the empowerment of women especially overseas; particularly in India and 3rd world countries and I'm still the same today. I was always very comfortable with going to the beach without a top on, I am very much for nipple equality. It never worried me who saw it to be honest, there are just boobs and I find it disgusting that we as a society sexualise boobs when there not actually a sexual organ, their meaning is quite beautiful which is of course breastfeeding.

I'm also big on equality, at one stage I looked at the empowerment of men as well especially with suicide and mental illness. I do believe that most likely men and women won't find equality, well probably not in my lifetime. It's a very negative statement I know, but I truly believe that's the reality of it. Due to so many withstanding factors such as culture, religion, stereotypes, pay gap, etc., finding that balance is going to be very hard and sad to say the least. I'm hoping we can create one small change in the world that can go onto creating bigger things or create a ripple effect and help benefit others lives or our grand childrens' lives; every single positive change helps!.

I struggled a lot with my faith, I was never really keen on the whole idea of religion to begin with, and I struggled to understand if there really was a god. I studied religion throughout high school and chose it as an elective subject in my final year of school. It was something I was very glad I did as it gave me so much knowledge and understanding of all religions.

I have to be honest it was through my studies that I came away from believing.

As I graduated the battle in my body was loosing, and I began to die slowly but oblivious to it all. I wish I knew my body so much more at this crucial time when it needed me to respond to it the most. I feel to this day I lacked an understanding of my own body. I didn't think any of this would ever happen to me and not a day goes by that I think back to the person I was then.

I really encourage everyone to get to know their body, listen to any changes, look for any warning signs; bodies are so amazing yet so flawed by nature. Only you know you're our own body best, when you feel like something is wrong or something doesn't feel right, don't ever put off getting it checked out! Don't put off anything in the way of your health, one day you could be thinking you're happy and healthy and the next you could be diagnosed with a disease, cancer or whatever it maybe!

You only have one chance, don't dwell on the small things and really cherish yourself. Cherish who you are and who you want to be not what others want you to be. Know your body; don't let anything or anyone stand in the way of your health and happiness.

Chapter Four
Radiation

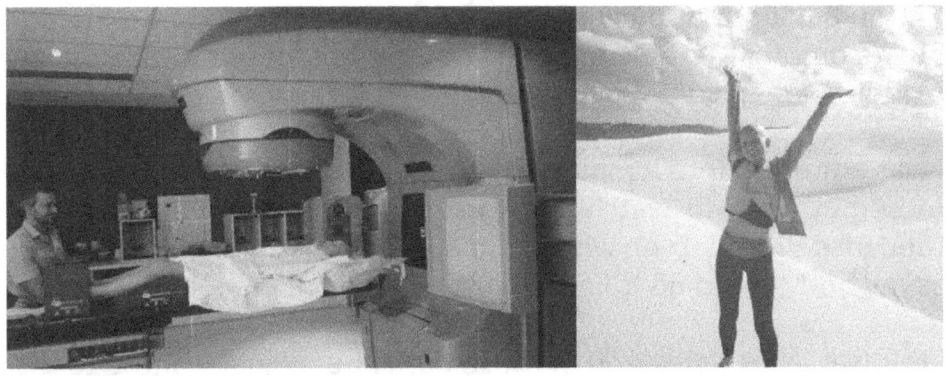

Leading up to radiation I thought it would be a breeze and wouldn't be as bad as chemotherapy, it only goes for 20minutes, I will be out the door in no time.

I walked into my first session thinking it would be easy, a walk in the park almost. I will later learn it was about to become one of the most painful and destroying experiences of my life.

During my radiotherapy treatment, I had to still keep having chemotherapy. In the first week of radiation, I was to begin a new chemotherapy drug called Irinoticane that I was to have once every day for an hour after radiation over a 5-day period. I was to do this again in the fourth week of my 6-week plan of radiotherapy treatment.

During my radiation treatment, my mum and I were so blessed and thankful to be offered a beautiful house to stay in called "Harry's House" at Stockton. A beautiful family own and run this house especially for cancer families. They had lost their beautiful son Harry at the young age of 6 to Neuroblastoma, and the house is named after their son.

Having this opportunity to stay in this wonderful house through such a horrible time is something I am truly beyond thankful for. Just having a 15-minute drive to and from the hospital instead of over an hour was just wonderful. We could go back to the house and I could sleep, as that's all I felt like doing.

Within a couple of days of having both radiation and Irinoticane I lost complete and utter control of my bladder and bowels, my kidneys were also beginning to fail.

I was admitted into hospital to have antibiotics and fluid and was to be put on 24hr watch and care. I couldn't eat, the thought of food made me ill. Even when I did eat I had to run to the bathroom, as my body could no longer digest or break down food properly.

I felt like I was dying and in those dark hours I just wanted to die, I felt useless, and like a child again, I couldn't even make it to the bathroom in time I just had no control whatsoever; by Saturday I had barely eaten for most of the week.

Due to the Irinoticane causing a very bad reaction, and as I was having radiation treatment, the doctors decided to stop this chemo drug and just keep going with radiation. Thank goodness!

When I got out of hospital I still hadn't recovered from the Irinoticane and I had only gained back little control of my bladder and bowels; just enough to make that few metres to the bathroom. I spent the rest of that weekend sleeping, crying and feeling dreadful.

My radiation doctor, Dr Kupta was one of the loveliest and down to earth men I had ever met. We saw him once a week during my time of having radiation treatment for regular checkups, questions and prescriptions. The radiographer team that I had were just as lovely and awesome to talk to; it always made my experience just a little bit better.

The time on the machine was a little longer than I thought, as I had two spots that needed to be zapped which was my pelvis and my fibular bone on my left leg. When you do radiation you don't feel a thing at the time of treatment, it's like an invisible force that enters your body, and you don't feel a thing.

It's hours after you get tired or feel side effects or permanent damage to the area being radiated.

After the first week of radiation and chemotherapy hell, the second and third week were okay, to say the least compared to the rest. I had experienced both issues with my bladder and bowel and not eating still. I slept constantly most days and was awake at the most for a couple of hours.

Staying where we were in Stockton really helped but I only ever saw the hospital and then back to the house and my bed. The house was only 5 minutes to Newcastle CBD by ferry and a street away from the beach. The only time I left the house was to go for treatment.

I really wanted to go outside; I stared out the window as much as I could to at least embrace the beauty of the garden and trees. I became that sick that leaving bed was just out of the question for me. I felt very isolated and lonely and felt very sorry for myself too. Those weeks of waking up, going to treatment, then back home and again and repeating over and over again began to feel monotonous, and I missed my friends, my own bed and being able to move or walk outside.

I lost a lot of weight quickly; my bones began to stick out of my chest, stomach and butt. My bones stuck out so much that it hurt to even sit down.

I began to look gaunt, very pale and dark circles began to appear around my eyes. I honestly looked like a bald witch and found it immensely hard to look at myself. I would even cry when I put on clothes that I loved, and they no longer fitted me.

The hospital began to threaten me with a feeding tube and gave me a drink called Ensure, one small popper which had over 400 calories in it, to get me to put on weight.

I was so determined to not get a feeding tube as feeding tubes are horrible and they make you look so much sicker; I definitely would have lost my self-esteem with a feeding tube.

During the third week of radiation treatment, my bowel and bladder issues grew worse, and my bladder felt like it was on fire. My pelvic area, bikini line and my left knee began to turn this awful red colour mixed with brown on the surface of the skin.

Even going to the bathroom or brushing my teeth seemed to become harder every day. My blood pressure would drop constantly, and I had a fear of collapsing in the shower so I tended to not have one every day for fear I'd hit my head. Radiation was destroying me from the inside out, and I spent days not eating. I just couldn't bring myself to even look at food, even if it was a favourite. There were some days I experienced random food cravings; one example was mashed potato, I don't know why but I just craved this type of starchy food.

I had many sleepless nights. I'd get up at least five times a night as my bowel and bladder were so inflamed. I became scared of going to the toilet as it was beyond agonising and it was only the third week, and I didn't think I could possibly go on any longer...

To ease the fear within myself of relapse and to also feel an accomplishment at the end I still desperately wanted to complete my 6 weeks of radiation treatment. At week three, my radiation doctor thought that I wouldn't even make it to week 5.

Dr Kupta did everything he could to help make it just that little bit more comfortable for me. There wasn't anything that I could do to ease the inflammation or being in constant agony when trying to go to the bathroom. I was given mainly very strong painkillers ranging from Endone to OxyContin. They helped me at least sleep and ease the pain from the third degree burns that were slowly appearing on my pelvis, bikini line, and leg area. He also gave me many topical creams and suggested using Sorbelene constantly.

She Will Always Carry On

The bedside table in my room looked like a chemist shop; there was little room to even place my phone on it!

Each and every day I could feel my body being destroyed over and over again, my hopes and dreams of that little percentage I was given from prognosis of ever having kids was shattered and had left me completely then. My heart was beginning to break, my vagina, pelvic and buttocks area became swollen, and the burns were unbearable. I stopped looking at myself by this stage.

I was in agony, 24hrs a day, and 7 days a week.

By the end of the week, I felt like a dead person walking and the night times were horrific. I'd be sitting on the cold hard bathroom floor at 4am, if I wasn't vomiting I was crying, and I started to lose my hope and willpower to live. I hated God, I couldn't understand why me as I'd done nothing to deserve this; this thought kept constantly going in my head over and over again.

The next day as I went in for radiation I sat quietly by myself on the couple of chairs that was outside the machine room. A lady was already sitting directly opposite me when I sat down. As I looked at this lady, I was confused as she looked perfectly healthy and normal, not someone who'd be having radiation.

Her necklace caught my eye, it was a chain with a large cross hanging from it. As I looked away, she looked up at me and said: "You will have children..." She said very abruptly "I had stage IV cervical cancer in my mid-twenties and the doctors said there was no possible way I would ever have children. I'm 49 years old now and have four beautiful children all with perfect pregnancies and all being perfectly normal and healthy babies. Now don't you give up, don't ever lose hope! God is with you always, you are never alone." She began to hold on tightly to the cross on her necklace, "Don't listen to the doctors girl, they can be wrong. Listen to yourself, and God.

Nobody else's opinion matters but yours..." Her husband then interrupted us as he walked out of the treatment room; he had bandages and glad wrap covering half his blood red burnt chest and neck.

"This is my husband; he is currently having 5 weeks of radiation treatment. He has throat cancer" she said.

The husband turned towards me and said "Hello!" with a great big smile on his face.

She then stood up, and they both wished me well and said their goodbyes, as they both walked down the corridor she then yelled back "don't you give up now, Maddy!"

I turned back and went to an immediate state of shock. I couldn't believe it, how did this woman know to say that and how did she know MY NAME? I had no obvious nametag hanging off me so how could this be? Did she hear the radiographer say my name or my mum even?

I will never forget her face, and from that day forward, not a day went by that I ever felt alone again. That was way to coincidental and weird to say the least! I believed again, what begun to be the worst day began to be okay. The rest of the day I cried, a lot!

I was taking the highest dosage of OxyContin, and it was knocking me out, and I began to rely on it every single night I went to bed.

That weekend my brother Justin and my mum's partner Anthony came up for the weekend. We had organised for all of us to go quad biking on the Stockton sand dunes. I pulled myself together to do it as it was something I really wanted to do and I needed to get out of the house.

I had about two V energy drinks that morning and laid off the painkillers as much as I could.

Once we arrived at the quad biking station, we were debriefed about riding them. As I stood there two minutes went by, and my blood pressure dropped suddenly. I began to feel nauseous and very fatigued. I had to sit down for about twenty minutes to pull myself together.

We proceeded to get on our quad bikes and had a small group with two other Americans and a middle-aged couple.

We made our way through a small bush track and came out to the dunes, and it honestly took my breath away.

The adrenaline was so full and so surreal that it took my pain away and made me forget about my reality and especially any pain. I remember just crying, it was that overwhelming.

I'm a strong believer in the healing powers of Mother Nature; the beauty of the world around us has healing powers within itself. The fresh air, the silence, the trees, the ocean, animal life, the sky that surrounds you has a lot of healing, take it all in and embrace it.

Even when you don't think you can do it or you don't think you can make it through those times, you can!! Put your mind to it and push yourself because you honestly can, it can be very empowering and the experience can change you and can be just what you needed.

After taking many photos at the top of the sand dunes and going nearly 100km an hour down sand dunes, breathing in the fresh ocean air it was over before I knew it.

It was back to reality and I as I got off the bike the pain immediately kicked back in, and I felt like vomiting.

Once back in the car I practically passed out, my body was that exhausted. I was on such a huge adrenaline high, but as my body returned to normality, I quickly started to feel my pain return.

When we arrived back home, I jumped into bed and slept for 16 hours straight.

It's now the second last week of radiation, week 5. My body felt destroyed, and I felt that there was no point in doing my daily mind activities or keeping positive within myself. I honestly thought my body could never repair itself ever again, it just felt so damaged. The days were meaningless and I was so drugged up on Oxycontin that I forgot what day it was.

I kept loosing more and more weight, and I was beginning to waste away. I began wearing loose track pants and baggy tops to hide it, and most of my other clothes no longer fitted me.

Looking at myself in the mirror made me very sad, I was losing myself and the body I knew. My boobs began to disappear (I always loved my boobs) and I had no curves. I also had a thigh gap, which was something that I would have wished for a year prior to my diagnosis and now I don't want, I hated it; it was so unnatural on my body. I had finally just learnt to accept and embrace my body before my diagnosis, and now I felt like it was being taken away from me.

Being thin, or wanting a thigh gap and being under your natural weight isn't fun and doesn't bring fulfilment at all.

Just love what you have, no matter what weight or size!! We don't know everybody's individual and personal pain when it comes to body confidence, so build yourself and everybody around you and not judge. All I wanted was my curves and boobs back. Eat what you want and not succumb to pressure and advertising.

My burns became increasingly more painful and turned into huge blisters. I really was determined to not give up on myself and life.

In the second last week of the radiation, I only did Monday to Thursday as it was the Easter long weekend.

She Will Always Carry On

My mum had planned to go up to Nelson's Bay only half an hour from Newcastle with a whole group of family friends. When we left on Friday morning, I felt lethargic and tired. My Easter spirit and my desire to want to eat chocolate that weekend didn't exist. The night before we left I cried and cried to my mum; I felt I could not go on anymore. I only had Tuesday to Thursday of the following week to do radiation but I felt I'd had enough, I felt it in my body, and my subconscious was telling me I was done.

My mum became worried she thought that if I didn't do it, it could be the difference between the cancer being destroyed or coming back. I didn't believe that fact at all, I felt it within myself that I'd given it my all and that it was okay to come to a certain point of thinking that's it, no more pain, no more devastation; I need to heal.

I understood my mum though, and where she was coming from, she just wanted to rid me of this disease; I just kept reassuring her of how I felt and how far I have actually now come.

Once at Nelson's Bay, I slept for basically the rest of the day until around dinnertime. When I got up, all of our family friends were squished into our little cabin lounge room drinking beers and chatting, it was a fun vibe.

They had cooked up an amazing smorgasbord of food, but I couldn't embrace that either. I so longed to be able to eat a normal meal.

The beach was about a 2-minute walk from the caravan park where we were staying. We all went down the next day as it was a very above average hot day, thank goodness one of the ladies had brought along a great big beach umbrella.

As I walked into the water, the saltwater was so painful on my burns, it hurt and stung like crazy. Saltwater has a lot of natural healing powers especially when it comes to skin and rejuvenating.

As the waves hit me back and forth I began to sob, not only was it painful around my pelvis, but I couldn't go under the water because of my central line; it was soul destroying.

By this point I was becoming more and more mentally drained, it was all beginning to tear me apart.

Arriving back at the cabin after the beach, I felt as if I'd run a five-day marathon, well at least that's what it felt like. Both the saltwater and sun had drained me and my pain began to get worse.

I'd never fully got the chance to look at the extent of my burns so I stood in front of the full-length mirror in my room.

My bikini and the insides of my vagina and buttocks area were completely burnt and had fully blistered. I looked like I had third degree burns and my skin had melted. Parts of my pelvis and mainly my bikini line began to turn a deep black colour; I began to shake, scream and cry. My mum and Anthony were out at the time on a walk, so I decided to just let it out all by myself.

For women it's one of the most sensitive and one of the worst parts of your body to ever have burnt; I sat in foetal position clinging to myself while crying. Nobody should ever have to go through this, not even my worst enemy. This was truly something else, radiation is a monster. It destroys you from the inside out. I am DESTROYED.

It was Easter Sunday, and we all took the ferry across to Tea Gardens from Nelson's Bay.

It was a perfect, warm and sunny day. We had all decided to stop and have lunch at the local pub. The majority of my time was spent in the toilet either vomiting or reapplying cream onto my burns. I just wanted to be by myself, I didn't want anybody to see me in the state I was in.

Talking to others and putting in the effort to have a conversation with someone became too exhausting for me.

Having to walk 50 metres back to the ferry wharf that afternoon was a massive effort for me. I had to sit down many times to pull myself back together and bring my blood pressure back up again. Once back at the cabin I lay on my bed and cried, I could not enjoy life or do anything anymore. Everything was beginning to become too much, too full, and I could no longer cope. The pain was never ending.

That evening I got a message from the girls, and they were driving up the next day to Stockton to catch up with me as I had not seen them for at least 5 weeks; it was definitely something that I needed. Annabelle, Hephzibah, Emily and Heather arrived about an hour after we arrived back at Stockton and I was very excited to see them.

I was feeling okay that morning for the first time in a long time. I had really wanted to go to one of the local beaches as one had a beautiful ocean bath which I could sit in.

Once the girls arrived, we all sat down on the lounge room floor, and we talked and talked.

It was hard for me deep down to come to terms with my situation as the girls talked about their lives at University, their jobs and going out: things I should be doing too.

When they asked me about what's been happening and how I have been, I didn't really want to tell them. I didn't want to talk about it, so I just told them the basics; even then their were faces filled with much despair. I immediately reassured them I was okay although I felt I was slowly fading away on the inside.

We left for the 15-minute drive to one of the local beaches called Merewether. When I took off my clothes down to my bikini, I remember seeing Hephzibah and Emily's faces of disbelief as they stared at my body. They both then immediately looked down in shock.

I never said anything about losing 6 kilos in a matter of 5 weeks, if they brought up anything to do with my weight I yet again reassured them that it happens with this treatment.

I am an open person and very honest, but sometimes I feel there are certain things that people shouldn't know or would be better of knowing when the time feels right.

The saltwater was painful against my body and this time I think it was worse. It honestly felt like a hundred needles being slammed into my skin all at once.

After a lovely day at the beach and catching up with the girls, they left that afternoon about 5pm. In the back of my mind, I was waiting for the conversation to come up with my mum about me stopping radiation but it never did; until the next day with the doctor.

As we sat quietly in the waiting room that Tuesday morning, my mum suddenly asked me to keep going even if it was just today. "Just one more!" She kept saying.

She really wanted me to do it for her, I didn't really understand why but she badly wanted me to.

I said "no mum! I'd had enough, you have seen the extent of my burns, and I am done. Dr Kupta didn't even think that I would get this far and I clearly have". I was very firm with mum about it and in the end, the decision was mine. I was very determined to say no, and I had a plan in my head of what I was going to say to Dr Kupta.

As Mum and I sat there discussing as to why I should and why I shouldn't, Dr Kupta walked out and called us in.

I knew doctors all too well by this point, and they are very sly and convincing in their own way to make you do things.

Once I finished explaining to Dr Kupta why I didn't want to continue and showed him my burnt pelvis, he very well understood me, yet he kept saying that I was here now and why not do just one more treatment.

I eventually gave in, but I well and truly did not want to do it.

As I walked into the treatment room and put on my gown, I began to fight back tears.

The radiotherapist put on an INXS cd as they knew I loved that band to help cheer me up.

They measured my pelvis, and all left the room, and the machine started. As it immediately began making its way around me I began to pray. I said "God, don't let this hurt me, I can't do this anymore! I'm DONE! Please help me..."

The machine made its way around to the top mark to line up with the bottom mark to shoot through the radiation and then suddenly the machine stopped.

As I laid there crying holding both my hands together one of the radiographers came over the intercom and said "Maddy, we're just going to restart the machine, we are not sure why it's doing this but re-booting the system will make it work again, sorry!"

They repeated this process four times and tried to run different tests to make it work, but the machine didn't budge.

I began crying hysterically, three of the radiographers walked in, and one said "we're so sorry Maddy, we are not sure what's wrong with the machine it hasn't done this before. We just spoke to Dr Kupta, and he said you should go home, as we know you have had a stressful day."

I walked out of the treatment room shaking never to return to that room again.

The idea that this state of the art radiation machine worth millions of dollars could just randomly stopped working is beyond powerful. Somebody had listened to me, I was so shocked, and I still get shocked months on when I re-tell this story.

I did return the next day just to see Dr Kupta and to have dressings put on my burns; it was my last appointment with Dr Kupta for at least 6 months. As we finished up, he handed me a box with a piece of paper and went on to explain about another side effect nobody had told me about.

He explained that when a woman has radiation on the pelvic area it shrinks the inside wall of the vagina and those muscles become lax. You need to use a dilator to work those muscles to push them back to their normal size.

If you don't use the dilator regularly, you will never be able to have intercourse, children or a proper gynaecology checkup.

This news shattered me and my coming into womanhood is now going to have even bigger issues; I felt I had been through enough and now this; it made me angry.

I left shattered... Sex isn't everything, but it does play a part in a relationship, all these thoughts and scenarios began to run through my mind. How do I explain this to another person?

Later that day we left Stockton to go home, and I was so excited to finally go back to my own bed and my own room. I was proud of myself for getting so far with my treatment, yet I still had this sadness inside as to what it did to my body.

I fell into my bed and didn't move for the next two weeks.

Two weeks after completing radiation treatment I ended up in the hospital with complications.

One morning I woke up with an enormous blister hanging from the right side of my vagina, a 40-degree temperature and abnormally fast heartbeat, I was immediately taken to the hospital.

I didn't realise but on the way to the hospital the blister popped and was oozing a lot of fluid.

It took a couple of days for my temperature to return to normal and as the burns tried to heal, it affected my walking. I was given constant fluids, dressing changes and antibiotics. I also noticed the skin on the left side of my vagina began to turn into a horrible colour of black.

This experience was beyond horrific.

After returning home for a week, I woke up during the night with a very painful intense throbbing in my right butt check. I took a painkiller to try and sleep, but the pain became unbearable, and mum took me to the hospital yet again.

They gave me a very high dose of morphine which knocked me out for most of the next day. After doing an ultrasound, the result was immense inflammation in the muscles of my left butt cheek, which was most likely caused by radiation. It thankfully did not develop into a cyst as they would have needed to conduct an operation to remove it. I spent the next week in hospital kept on heavy painkillers; all I did was sleep, I didn't even know what day it was when they discharged me.

Since radiation, I have never been able to go to the bathroom the same.

I struggle to digest food and have irritable bowel. My peripheral nerves in my left leg have been affected by radiation and I can't place my foot fully on the ground. I started having physio and was given a boot to wear. I also think about what I would do if I meet somebody and my pelvic area is definitely not the same.

The effects of radiation will haunt me for the rest of my life, and I worry about long-term side effects. I still tell myself that I've achieved a lot and through all the pain and agony I suffered, I never gave up!

Chapter Five
Spiritual Healing & Strategies

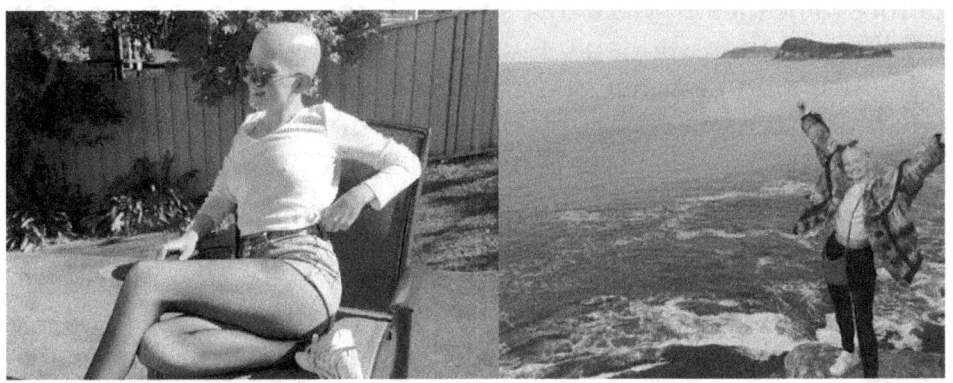

I would never take back my cancer or any of the tough times for I wouldn't be where I am today as a person spiritually, mentally, physically and emotionally; we are shaped by tough times and life experiences.

When I was first diagnosed, I was very angry, and it definitely made me turn against anything that I ever believed in.

One day I was at the local shopping centre and a woman just came up to me suddenly and said "I feel like I'm being pull towards you and that I need to say this to you. God is healing you, he is with you. Whether you believe it or not, you are being healed and the earth is healing you. " She then prayed for me.

At the time I was very freaked out and didn't think too much of it.

Days after I suddenly realised that there was no point in being angry with my illness or the world anymore, I wanted to move forward. I felt at this time I needed to pray, look to nature and become very mindful. I wanted to believe that if I died, I'd go to a good place although at times I felt stupid praying.

I'm a strong believer of purpose and feeling, and that everyone has a purpose in life. I believe every human being on this earth is given a purpose, no matter how big or small; everybody is here for a reason, especially you!

Before my cancer I was a lost soul and struggled for a purpose in my life and then suddenly I was diagnosed with cancer and had a big wake up call that was to change my life forever. Whether you have had your wake up call already or still waiting, know and believe that you will. Search for it, of course, it doesn't have to be cancer or health related. Travel, try new things, change your job it could be any of those, and you may not realise that it could be standing right in front of you.

Be open to change, never lose faith, at the time it may not feel like it will ever get better but believe me it will because miracles do happen and things can work out. When I was diagnosed and given that 4% chance of making it through, I looked at that number and resounded "that 4% is going to be me".

Without those hard times you have been through in your life you wouldn't be who you are today. Embrace change, watch documentaries, fill yourself with worldly perspectives and you could begin a whole new journey with life and meaning.

POWER OF THE MIND:

The mind is everything!

It can destroy you, bring you unhappiness and uncertainty. Or it can bring you fulfilment, positivity and happiness.

I created a mindset of just trying to keep positive and focus on my goal, even during the horrific days of radiation it always sat at the back of my mind keeping me grounded. I never let go of that thought.

There are better days ahead!! Grab those amazing moments and good days and always know there will be many more of those to come in your life.

In the western world we have a lot of mental illness, if you look at the 3rd world countries there isn't as much, why?

Is it that some countries are poor and underprivileged and don't have the wealth of the western world? Is it that they take everything they can, embrace what they have and try to live out their lives as much as they can? They appreciate the smaller things more and have so much more faith and appreciation. In certain places, they also have a very strong sense of faith and culture.

It's like the more you have, the more you want and the richer you want to be. This mindset can sometimes not be such a good thing for your mental health and wellbeing. In the western culture, we look to materialistic things to bring us satisfaction, but it's only temporary. Stereotypes, body shaming, gender expectations, media and technology are becoming out of control, from day one we are drilled with the more prettier, richer and powerful you are the more happier and fulfilled you will been in your life.

Everyone needs to stop and realise that what they have is amazing and every day is a blessing. Eating healthy food three times a day, having your mum there with you or having children are all a blessing as others may not experience that anymore or may never will.

Look at your life and current situation from a worldly point of view, don't be a slave to society, start being your own person and be happy with what you have. Search for meaning and put yourself out there!

We are taught to dislike ourselves and not be satisfied with how we look at anything toxic that the media and society have taught you, you can unlearn it. There are no genes that are given to you from birth for having self-hatred, negativity, sexism and racism we are all one.

YOU can only help yourself before others can help you, ignore societies standards, people's opinions and only listen to yourself.

The power is within you.

One day you can be here and the next you could be gone.

After my diagnosis I thought I am not going to stop living, this cancer is not going to take everything from me

I lived each day as best as I could and learnt to understand that it's okay to cry and have bad days. Of course, there are going to be bumps and bad weather on your journey through life, but that's what life is all about. In the spectrum of things it's only small and temporary, don't let your tough times or illnesses ever control you!!

Mind is key.

SAFE SPACE AND MIND HEALING:

My safe space was my room, kind of typical of a teenager but a safe space could be anything! Having your own safe space to be alone and heal is vital.

In my safe space, I relax, read, write, meditate and listen to music; it helps me zone out.

- I do it mostly everyday and I while I do it I sometimes would just listen to my breathing.
- I do a lot of guided meditations, most from online or sound cloud, it helps me calm myself.
- I would create these visuals in my mind of imagining positiveness being sent from my brain and everywhere in my body straight to my tumour. I'd image the tumour being destroyed and my beautiful, healthy green cells having a party. I'd do it for about 5-10minutes, and the images did change from time to time, I imagined the positive and negative cells and the tumour itself. I believe nature has a strong force against cancer; I truly believe that I can help undo the cancer naturally through my mind and a good healing space.

- During chemotherapy, I would image my body to be this shiny, beautiful green light and everything flowing beautifully. Helping blocked energy to be freed and imagining the chemotherapy itself going straight to the tumour and destroying it for good!

THE HEALING POWER OF HANDS:

Hands are a beautiful healing power, filled with a lot of energy.

Every day I would put both my hands on the top area of where the tumour was. I would listen to my breathing and constantly thinking of my positive thoughts over and over again. . I normally did this when I was relaxed, most of the time before bed.

I don't believe in others putting their hands on me while praising the Lord or believing they can heal because I believe I can heal myself.

The healing power is within you, I don't think it's necessary for others to heal me, it's my body and I know what feels right.

RID YOURSELF OF ALL NEGATIVITY AND LET GO OF PAST TRAUMAS:

To have a positive mindset, you need to let go of your past traumas and suffering. If you hold on and store negativity you don't help yourself or your mind at all.

I immediately let go of my past traumas and forgave all the people who hurt me. I read up on this article about a way of doing it, and I swear it was the most amazing thing to come into my life.

In my head I imagined myself sitting at a campfire around a bright fire with people around me who represent a past trauma, suffering, bad experience, personal problem, etc.

Each day I would visit it in my head, and I would go up to each person individually, and I would imagine myself forgiving them and hugging them and as I hugged them the person disappeared in my arms. One by one all the people who were sitting around me in my campfire would disappear until it was just me, just myself being in a beautiful place, being mindful and at peace. It took about a week for me to finish this exercise in my head as a couple of times I would go back to the fire, and somebody who I thought I forgave and let go off had reappeared again, meaning I hadn't forgiven or let go the first time.

Rid yourself of negative people; don't let anyone bring you down especially when you're in a time of need or going through a rough patch in your life.

Find an understanding within yourself to not get frustrated at times when you feel nobody understands your pain or what you're going through. Talk to people who listen, talk out your anger and feelings; never hold it in because it's not good for your body. Often, people want to do things for you even if you don't want them to, so let them, it makes the other individual feel happy and fulfilled.

NATURAL ALTERNATIVES AND CRYSTALS:

I did my fair share of research on other natural medicines and plants that can help with destroying cancer and being cured.

When doing so, you need to be careful as there is a lot of inaccurate sources out there on the deep wide web.

Like I said before about frankincense and black cumin seed oil, each had a lot of resources and stories to back it up. I also found a lot on alkaline water and that drinking it can cause cancer to die, as they can't live in an alkaline positive environment.

- Shop around for 100% frankincense, there is a lot around that are not pure. I would apply about 3-4 drops to the area where my cancer was while doing my hand healing and positive thoughts in believing this is helping.
- Black cumin seed oil once a day. A tablespoon of it with a teaspoon of honey to help you swallow it and it tastes better.
- I drank as much alkaline water as I could, sometimes it did get expensive; so try and buy in bulk.

Somebody suggested I look into crystals as they have a lot of healing powers and can help with anger.

I researched about what types of crystals were out there. I was particularly drawn to amethyst with its powerful attributes relating to health and wellbeing. I always held my amethyst necklace and key chain close to me especially during days of chemotherapy, radiation and when I was struggling mentally. I also held it in my hands when I prayed believing it was giving me strength.

One day I was reading a magazine, and it had a great big article on the powers of Himalayan rock salt lamps in your home and bedroom. I went and bought one and put it beside my bed. My previous lamp was bright, but rock salt lamps are dim and give a good sense of relaxation and good energy for your room.

"Cancer is formed by nature and I feel within myself that through natural things such as rocks and medicines from the earth, they can help undo one's cancer and can help in the process of one day finding a cure. Doing it is one thing, but truly believing in the healing remedies of the earth is a whole different level."

– Maddy Ritchie

MEDICAL MARIJUANA:

I myself am a firm believer of medical marijuana, I didn't always take it, but definitely throughout radiation and at the beginning it helped ease my nausea and calmed me down.

Medical marijuana was always my immediate option if all my other options were exhausted or if my cancer were to relapse.

If you are someone that suffers from extreme nausea from medication or treatment, I would highly recommend it. Just know that all bodies are different and may slightly differ in how well it can help you.

I do to an extent believe it helped on my path in trying to beat cancer; I wouldn't say it has cured it but definitely helped my body with pain.

THE FOOD DILEMMA:

From day one I was drilled with constant opinions from people and certain doctors about "eating healthy" or "don't go near that food" and "Sugar fuels cancer"

EAT WHAT YOU WANT! I ignored everyone's ridiculous opinion as I myself don't believe it fuels my cancer. I'm not saying to eat bad foods all day every day, there were days I never ate at all but to put weight on I needed some sugar and fat in my diet; even my dietician agreed.

Some days after chemotherapy I ate Mac Donald's as I craved it badly and a month later I was cancer free on my scans.

Of course, food plays a big part in your healing process and eating well is of course a good thing, but cutting out sugars and fats, etc. is not necessarily the answer.

Throughout most of my treatment, I listened to my body, satisfied my cravings and tried to eat in moderation.

We have all these ridiculous ideas and myths towards food and I myself ignored it all and listened.

You can go through your whole life constantly eating healthy and keeping fit but still get cancer or major health problems.

I'd led a fit and healthy life prior to my cancer and never would have thought I'd get cancer.

I will never forget one day when I was on a bus, and a woman sat down next to me and started talking to me she said " I was in my 50's and I was diagnosed with bowel cancer, and I had no genetic inheritance in my family. I never smoked, never drank alcohol and constantly ate healthy for my whole life up and then got bowel cancer. My brother ate junk food, drank alcohol, smoked all his life and the bastard is nearly 90 years old in a fit condition..."

Cancer does not discriminate and don't ever fear food!

NATURE:

Being out and embracing nature is a very good way to be by yourself for healing and meditating. Just being thankful for the world and environment that surrounds you is very healing. From day one of diagnosis I looked at my surroundings and realised how much I took it for granted, I began to embrace it during tough times and I really adored being outside.

Learn to love nature and the environment your in, sit outside as much as you can and take it all in and enjoy the fresh air we breathe.

Chapter Six
Relationships & Stigmas

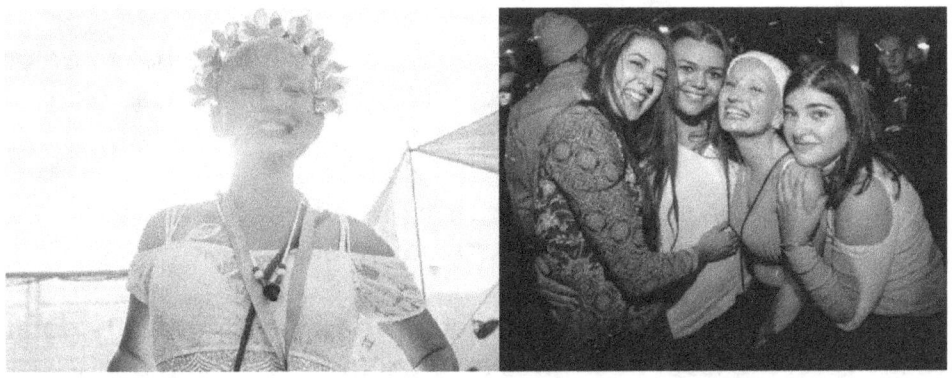

Cancer can of course bring tough times but can also bring about unwanted problems when it comes to relationships and also family matters.

I ended up cutting all ties with Mr X the week after radiation finished and I immediately felt free and so much happier. Due to the effects of radiation and not being able to have intercourse this became a big bone of contention for Mr X and that was it for me. I also felt that I could and do deserve better and deserved to be valued and respected more.

I grew and changed as a person during my treatment and said goodbye to both him and people that didn't mean anything to me in my life; things changed for me.

It was hard to deal with at first but learning to just be on my own was one of the best things that happened.

I learnt more about myself losing people in my life during that time than in my whole entire life.

I forgave Mr X pretty quickly after we broke up as all I wanted to do was move on. I honestly hoped to never see him again and chose to not hold onto any negativity for him, in fact, I wanted to thank him for making me a stronger person.

He couldn't handle the breakup and I could sense a few other people couldn't either, a lot of people didn't know what to do or how to act around me anymore, and I learnt that it was okay. I didn't quite understand why they changed towards me.

If somebody can't be with you through the good and bad times, then they don't deserve to be with you at all.

I'm not sure where Mr X has ended up now, and I honestly don't really care, the last I heard was he'd taken the breakup badly.

I do honestly hope the best for him in life and that he finds happiness.

When I was first diagnosed people that weren't even friends or ever spoke to me at school decided it would be a good time to become my friend. I'm not sure whether it was for them to feel better about themselves, to look good or whether they genuinely did care about my illness and me. I tried to just ignore it as to me they were far from genuine, especially the ones who said horrible things about me at school. It didn't make any sense to me and didn't ever bother me too much, I just took it for what it was and thanked them for their support.

When I was first diagnosed it was when everyone began to move on from school life to adulthood and university. Some of my friends fully moved on and never spoke to me again and some, of course, stuck around and helped me through this journey.

I struggled immensely as I did sometimes feel I was being left behind and held back by this disgusting thing called cancer. I know though that one day it will be me, I always told myself that I will be normal again and that I can achieve these things but just not right now.

I became very distant with a lot of my friends as we all changed as individuals and they did their own thing.

I did struggle with loneliness and felt very isolated and really wanted a friend to relate to and lean on in those dark times. I had my mum and she was wonderful, and we did talk a lot but just to have a special girlfriend to talk about other things like boys. I am very thankful for a few girlfriends that did stick by me and visited me in the hospital, they are the ones I cherish the most.

I was always honest with my girlfriends about how I felt and whether I needed to go home, felt unwell or about what I was going through. It's my reality, and I wasn't afraid to share it with them as that's what friends are for.

The relationship between my mum and me has brought us closer together from day one of diagnosis. She is both my mother, my carer and my friend and she is also the one that struggles with my cancer the most (and still does). I think I honestly coped better than her and was quicker accepting it than she was.

She gave up her job to care for me and has sacrificed a lot. Being together at times drove us both a little crazy, but nothing ever came between us.

I relied on her a lot (and still do) and some days I felt like a 10-year-old. I felt I couldn't be without her when I stayed in the hospital; I needed my mum there. She never was a fan of Mr X, and she always knew that he did try to turn me against my own family at times (but that's another story).

My mum worries the most out of all my family, we try to keep equal balance between each other to have our own time and do our own things. She has only been with her partner Anthony for three years, and they still need time together to do things. I was concerned about her getting sick from worry as I've heard that carers can suffer the most when caring for a loved one when they feel so helpless. I always wanted to keep strong for her as it hurt me to know that she wanted to take the cancer from me and give it to herself.

Dealing with other people and their own stigmas towards cancer, stereotypes and opinions is something you really just have to ignore.

In the world we live in today, with social media everybody literally knows what you are doing or what you have been up to.

A lot of people associate with cancer that the individual is constantly in bed, sick, vomiting, doesn't do much.... Well you're wrong when it comes to expecting that from me!

Yes there can be people out there who deal with it like that, and of course, I have had my bad days, but it isn't bad all the time.

Everybody's body reacts differently depending on the treatment schedule and type of cancer.

I chose to live my life as much as I could and as best as I could from day one of diagnosis and this stupid idea that we just lay in bed and do nothing is stupid.

Our society is very judgemental so do what makes you happy not what other people's thoughts, opinions and what you "should" be doing in effect is trying to live your life to the fullest.

A lot of people expected me to be at home the whole time and one day when I said I had been to the beach some people just told me straight out "you shouldn't be doing that!" ummm can't I live my life? Or at least try to be normal, I sat under an umbrella for goodness sake!

Honestly, I just learnt to live my life on my own terms and how my body was feeling on the day or at that moment. I think I knew better than anybody else. I just learnt to ignore opinions and do what I felt like doing, I just wanted that normality.

Another stigma and expectation of a cancer patient is to wear a wig and not walk around bald.

I don't think I've ever worn a wig in my life, they are irritating and annoying. I always felt I didn't want to hide my reality and I just honestly didn't care about other people's opinions.

I really embraced who I was and understood that life is too short for this kind of bullshit. Learning to be comfortable in your own body is seriously the key to happiness. I never saw a point in hiding my bald head as this was my reality and I think I rocked a bald head!

One day I was at the local shopping mall and a woman in her late 60's came up to me and decided to just let me know "Whoa! You walked out of your house bald! I wouldn't even dare to do that" well, old woman you must be living in the time zone of 1945.

I just looked back at her with piercing eyes and said: "Sorry what?" There was no point in fighting this woman as she was obviously stuck in the most ridiculous mindset.

I just walked away and thought to myself how dare you say that? How dare anybody say that!

There is a lot of inequality about the awareness of cancer and differences in cancer funding.

People straight away presume that I have breast or cervical cancer because there seems to be more awareness of these cancers. I deserve people to understand my cancer and not look at me strangely when I tell them its name. I'd like to see people understand there are a lot of childhood cancers that are just as important and life threatening. Maybe this is part of my journey to educate and make people more aware of the different types of Rhabdomyosarcoma.

One example was a huge Australian bakery that did a breast cancer fundraiser and sold pink finger buns. Why was there not a yellow finger bun fundraiser to support childhood cancer?

Don't get me wrong I think it's a wonderful idea and I have nothing against breast cancer, but every cancer should be treated equally, and knowledge is power. It frustrates me that only 4% of funding goes to childhood cancer.

Cancer is cancer!!

I am a firm believer of education, it's the key, start teaching kids from primary school about the different types of cancers and how important it is to know your body.

At least one person dies every day from this insidious disease; we need to work together to one day find a cure!

All cancers deserve to be equal!

Chapter Seven

The News

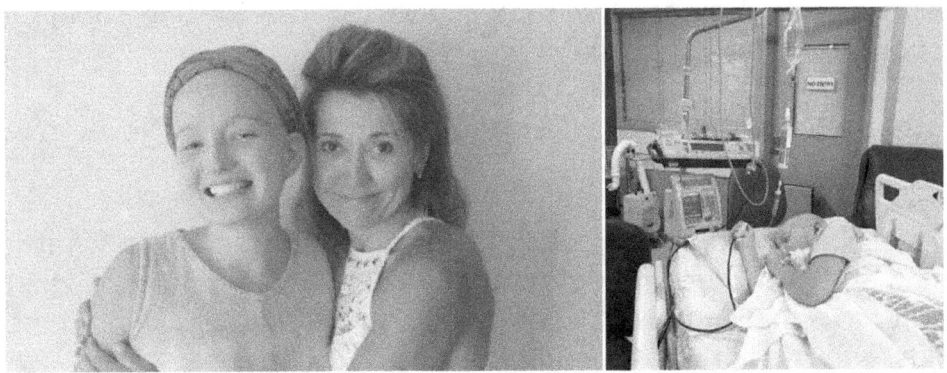

After the devastation and horrible offsets from radiation, I was becoming mentally exhausted. The treatment was beginning to take its full toll on me emotionally and mentally, and it began to be unbearable to cope.

What was helping me stay afloat was my determination to begin again after Mr X and find out new things about myself. For quite some time I held anger inside towards him but as time went on it honestly just faded away, and I started to enjoy being single.

I learnt from it and holding onto negative feelings wasn't going to help me in my getting through this treatment. I know I'll meet someone again and it will be the right time and place.

I became the stronger person in the end, and I came out winning!

After the 6 weeks of radiation treatment, I began chemotherapy again before the second round of scans.

I went out to dinner one evening with a few friends from school, and we went to a Chinese restaurant. It was the weekend before I had to do my gruelling week in the hospital for chemotherapy and I can honestly say I was a mess. I broke down in front of them all, I could no longer control myself or my emotions, and I just let it all out.

At the end of dinner the waiter gave us all a fortune cookie, I opened mine, and it said;

"Your tough times now will make up for your future, Never give up."

I sat in shock for a couple of seconds, I couldn't believe what it said and how much it applied to my life, and it felt like a sign. I still have that piece of paper beside my bed, just to remind me now and then of what it said.

The world works in such crazy ways, and I know someone must be looking out for me.

Due to the power of the Internet and my posts I was asked to do some public speeches throughout my local area at high schools or charity events; they were so rewarding.

I thought I'd be very confident as it was a lot harder than I thought talking about my cancer. The first time I was a wreck but as I did another speech I improved hugely and found my confidence. It really didn't bother me talking in front of a large crowd as throughout both primary and high school I was on debating team and did public speaking.

I also received a huge amount of support and feedback which truly filled me with such great joy.

It helped me believe again.

On the Sunday, a day before scan day, mum and I hosted a Biggest Morning Tea for cancer at our house. Lots of family and friends came, and the food was unbelievable, it was a huge success. We raised just over $1000 half of which went to the cancer council and the other half to the Kids Cancer Project. It was just awesome!

Leading up to the second round of scans bought on a lot of mixed emotions but with a great sense of accomplishment.

I felt well within myself and truly believed the scans would be better than the last and have no signs of the tumour.

My mum was of course worried and on edge and not thinking as positive as me.

I was very anxious for a few days before the scans, and I didn't sleep much as my brain would not switch off.

I really tried hard to have positive thoughts but honestly, those thoughts would creep into my thinking and you do have your questionable freak out moments of "oh shit, what if I'm wrong?" "Has it spread?" "Should have I done this or that differently?" I did that many times but tried to push that aside and focus on myself and really trust my body and how good I was feeling.

I had gone from having a tennis ball sized tumour to the size of a little pea and had an 80% chance of relapse.

Scan day came with a lot more emotion than I thought. I don't know why but I broke down when I was on the machines. I guess I was just very overwhelmed with emotions and scared. I did some slow breathing techniques to help calm me down but within a few hours I'd be a mess again.

I was due to stay in hospital that evening, and I would also be able to get my results that afternoon. All my family sat and waited in my hospital room eating leftover food from our Biggest Morning Tea.

Dr Alvaro arrived at 5pm with a huge big grin on his face and immediately gave us the results.

"The scans looked really good Maddy. There is no sign of anything remaining from the tumour; however, there is a great deal of muscle changes in and around the area. Which is to expected from your protocol and also because there was an 8cm tumour originally there."

I couldn't say anything, I just sat there speechless.

I immediately thought "Yeah that's right... I bloody knew it!!"

I wanted to laugh and cry at the same time, Frank smiled and said "No words huh? That's okay! Everything is good"

Yet with cancer there is a bad side to it, Frank went on answering my mum and dad's questions, which wasn't very pleasant to hear.

My dad asked, " So it will be over in October? And what would happen if it did relapse?"

Dr Frank said "Yes we still keep going until October with a finish date mid October and then onto maintenance tablets. In a worst case scenario if relapse happens between now and then or after October it would most likely be terminal and in some cases may not be treatable"

I had heard the worse case scenario before, and I hated hearing it again, I understand you have to prepare and be told the worst to have an idea of what's to come and also for Dr Frank to protect himself; but the scenario is awful.

I'm not afraid of death, I believe if it's my time to go then it is! There is nothing I can do about it. If that scenario were to arise, I know that I did everything I could and I will be in a place of peace watching over my family.

It felt like a weight was lifted off my shoulders. Dad, Anthony and Justin left not too long after while mum behind to make sure I was okay.

At 6:30pm that evening the nurse put up my chemo and within a couple of hours I was vomiting like crazy.

I didn't know now if it was due to my chemo being given every 3 weeks now or the chemo drug itself but oh God it was awful.

I was given a tablet for nausea, and this tablet helps you sleep too, I immediately fell asleep mentally and physically exhausted from such a big day.

The next day I ate nothing, watched Dr Phil and random documentaries while falling in and out of sleep. Justin arrived that afternoon at about 5pm and boy I was glad to see him, the day was insanely long and slow and by this time I was hungry and wanted to go home to my bed.

My 24hr maintenance fluids finished at 6:45 and I was gone by 7pm.

We stopped at a Mac Donald's on the way home, and I ate a whole big mac! How I did, I honestly I don't know.

Once home I fell into bed and passed out while listening to my music.

Chapter Eight

FROM ANOTHER PERSPECTIVE

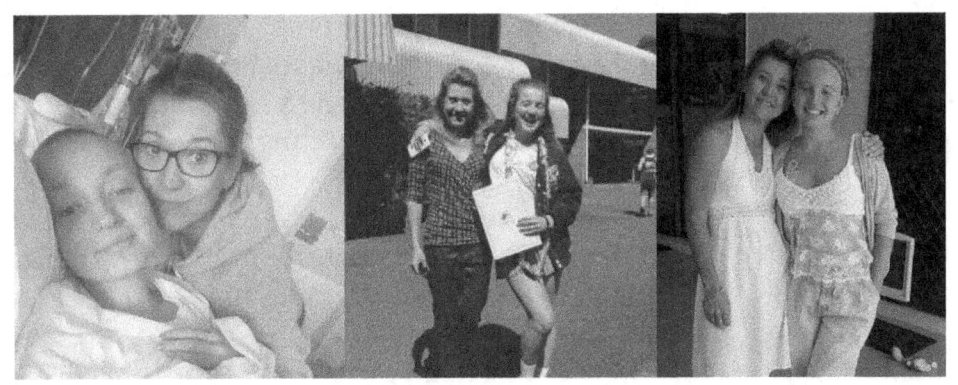

A Mother's Perspective: By Barbara Montgomery (Mum)

I've thought about what to write for Madison many times now. She asked me to write about how I felt with her diagnosis and the last 11 months. That little fear that sits in the pit of my stomach will never go away, and the fear that this disease can relapse will always be there. I try to push that fear away and keep positive, especially for Maddy. The bond between a mother and child will never be broken and to watch your child go through what Maddy has been through is so very heartbreaking. Yes, I've asked God why many times and still don't understand why she has been chosen to go on this journey. She is an amazing girl with the most beautiful smile. Is the journey for her to teach others to not take life for granted? I know it has made me stop and think of how life can change in the blink of an eye.

The date October 12th, 2015 will forever be embedded in my brain. At 10.30pm the surgeon informed us of an 8cm tumour in Maddy's pelvis. Shock, fear, pain what do you feel when your 17-year-old daughter has just been diagnosed. I never slept that night just cried and cried. The fear of losing my daughter just swirled in my head, and I couldn't let that fear go.

I spent hours researching Rhabdomyosarcoma, Alveolar, a name that I'd never heard but certainly do now. Research has improved over the years but still a lot more is needed to understand why a cell goes rogue. Still, the same question circling in my head WHY MADI?

The aggressive chemo Maddy had was too hard for me to watch at times, I would often leave her room for a minute to have a cry and then come back with a smile. So many times I wanted to take her pain away and make her feel better, I guess I felt a little useless, but she would be happy if I just stayed in her room overnight, which I always did. Not having hospital food made her extremely happy so I would often make us something yummy and still do.

I bless every day that I spend with Maddy and will fight this disease with all my being. Maddy deserves a beautiful life like we all do. I believe only God knows what's in store for us all.

We spent a week in Yulara (Northern Territory) at Sails Desert Resort thanks to the amazing people at the Starlight Foundation. I got to understand just how difficult it is for Maddy and the effect of the Vincristine chemo drug that has affected her left leg. She struggles to walk very far, and her energy levels are still very low. It was amazing to see Uluru (Ayers Rock) & Kata Tjipta (The Olgas) it seemed to have a very spiritual feeling for all of us. We found people to be very kind and giving when they found out about Maddy's treatment in the last 10 months. We got to do dinner under the stars, helicopter ride over the whole area, camel sunset tour and Kings Canyon. So many wonderful memories to keep and of course all the fabulous photos to treasure; not to mention staying in a lovely resort and having a car to drive around in.

We'd arrived back home, and I happen to see a young girl had passed away from Stage 4 Rhabdo. I then can't help but to wonder about this girl and her family and how difficult it must be for all of them and try to understand why she couldn't be saved.

On the happier, side I then read of another girl who has returned to high school and is playing soccer and looks amazing. My heart wants that girl to be Maddy too.

After reading Michael Crossland's book anything is possible. His story is truly inspirational. I could relate to the feelings his mother went through when Michael was on his journey. He has touched so many people. I'm hoping Maddy can do the same with her cancer story.

We've never had any cancer in our family only a history of heart problems. My father died of a massive heart attack at the front door of the family home. He had many heart issues over the years but seemed to always bounce back unfortunately not that last time. I know Maddy's brother Justin feels a lot of sadness inside although he doesn't say much. I think Justin and Maddy have grown a lot closer since the diagnosis and I know Justin would be there for Maddy in a second.

My partner Anthony has been such a support for me. He gets me to look at issues differently and tries to stop me stressing. I am a stressful person, and I think this journey has made me a little worse. He is very spiritual and believes in a higher power. To be honest, I'm not sure where I stand on the whole God thing. I still do say a prayer though in the hope that there is someone listening. Anthony & I have music in common with our duo; it's given me an outlet and taken my mind off everything even if it's just for a few hours. You have to try and stay in the normal routine as much as you can. There is depression in our family, and there has been a lot of times I could go easily go to that dark place, but I pull myself together and remember I need to be there for Maddy.

Maddy's Oncologist Dr Frank Alvaro and his team at John Hunter Hospital have always shown great support to Maddy, and I can't praise them highly enough. The nurses have been so wonderful and do such a fantastic job.

It must be so tough for them to see the children and teenagers going through these terrible diseases and to then loose some of them. I know Maddy hates being in hospital but now she only stays for one night, and that's so much more bearable for her.

We found a wonderful lady Naomi Sirio (SoulJourn) specialising in women's health, and she has been such a support to myself and to Maddy. She has been doing spiritual healing with Maddy, and I have gone to her for counselling. It's just another way to help us through this journey.

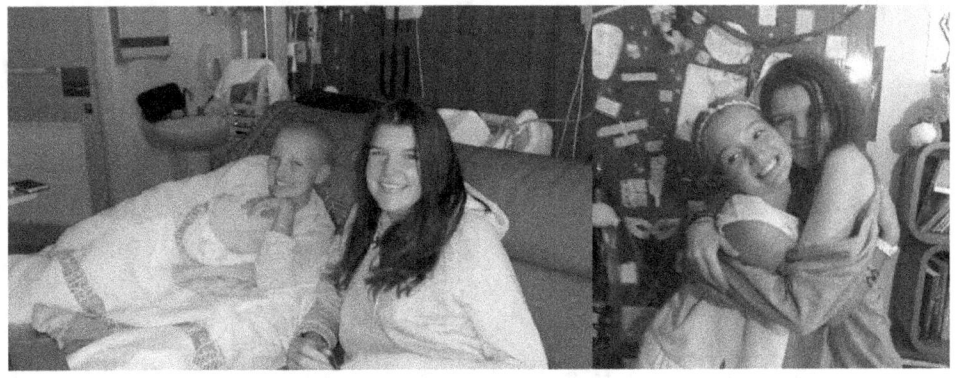

A Friends Perspective By Emily Willis (Close Friend)

It was October 2nd, 2015, the music was playing; we were laughing sitting around after spending the day in the sun and sand, talking about boys and our hopes and aspirations for the future. Summer was around the corner, and I was spending the weekend at my house with a few of my favourite girls Maddy and Vonnie. It was as normal as any other weekend, unaware that our naive, ignorant answers would postpone and grow a life changing event.

Friday evening we were getting changed into our bikini like any other time, swapping tops and trading bottoms when Maddy mentioned she had a bruise appearing around her bikini line, yellow and purple with a lump on the inside, confused about its origin but excited for the weekend ahead we all shrugged it off thinking it would disappear of its own accord at only 17 years of age, thinking we were all indestructible no one would think it to be cancer. I tell you the beginning of the story to emphasise the normality of our life, we are like any other teenagers in existence, excited for the next weekend dreaming of traveling the world and working out our lives in ignorance that it will not be the ordinary 9-5 and we will make an impact on the rest of the world.

The fact that my best friend was diagnosed with stage four cancer is not one that anybody could have foreseen or would even think had existed

Eventually, I knew things were not ok, I knew that there was a chance that oddly coloured bruise could be cancer but I will never forget the moment I was told she had been diagnosed. I was sitting on my bed when my mum came into my room, "I just got off the phone with Maddy's mum" she said and proceeded to tell me that she had stage four cancer, it had wrapped around her lower intestine, bowel and... she would be having chemo theory and then a potential operation. As the tears came to my eyes, I curled up onto my bed and cried.

I knew she was not going to die, there was no chance she was, she's way too strong and way to defiant for that. I knew that it was going to be hard and that we would not be prepared for what was to come.

I remember one of the first things she said to me upon her diagnosis "the cancer doesn't control me I control the cancer" and that was exactly how she's lived!

Being told your friend has 3 months to live, spending her 18th birthday seeing her go from having beautiful long blond hair to short inch dusty brown and having tubes coming out of her chest there is no words to describe it, but no matter what she might look like on the outside, to me she hasn't changed at all she is still the same funny, excited beautiful girl she has always been.

Seeing your friend in chemotherapy for the first time could be possibly one of the hardest things I have faced.

Being raised in a healthy middle-class family, having little exposure to illness from close family and friends and then to walk into a bland hospital room seeing the girl with who a few weeks prior you were at the beach with is something I wish upon no one.

It can bring you to tears and the struggle not to cry and burden your friend is a different matter entirely.

I remember the first time I visited the hospital I approached the door peering through the glass with a pain in my chest of heartache, plastering a smile on my face hoping Maddy couldn't see the pain. I entered with all words lost from my voice, but as soon as Maddy opened her mouth and started talking it was like life was breathed into the room, and not one thing had changed.

Maddy is the same girl she has always been! People look and treat her differently and assume her illness restricts her. On a small scale yes this is true, at the beginning of her treatment and during radiation her physical capabilities were somewhat impaired however her spirit and personality have forever remained the same.

To see people treat your friend differently, stare at her or approach her with fear or worry almost brings me to tears. I want to tell you that she is no different from you and me, although it is understandable to be sensitive about the issue. It breaks my heart to see her been treated any differently or approached with anxiety and to have people shine her like a prize for their own "popularity" as they did at the beginning of her diagnosis is frankly horrible. People do not stop living because they are diagnosed with cancer! This is an issue I cannot stress enough!

Maddy is exceptionally strong, and the most passionate optimistic girl I have ever met, but the fact that people associate her illness with limitations to life and changes to her personality is a myth that our media-filled society promotes and a theory that needs to become extinct.

I have seen her date, laugh, go to concerts, take spontaneous road trips, go to the beach and clubs and our society condones or judges this otherwise normal adolescent behaviour purely because she has been given one of the hardest things life can throw.

My message to anyone who is reading this is simple, people don't stop living, they don't change so please do not treat them differently, stare or associate any illness with a limit to how they want to live their own life

When dealing with the emotions that come from this situation, it is important to rely on your friends and others that are in the same position. I always made it a point never to cry in front of Maddy, on her 18th birthday I lasted the entire day without crying but as soon as I said goodbye and the door closed, I hadn't even walked down the stairs before I was sobbing. It's ok to cry, it's important to face the emotions, and it's better to embrace them than run from them. You're not the important one in this situation she is, and she's the one who needs you and the one who has it a million times harder. In this situation, I survived by talking to others who understand and for me that was my/her friends, Hephzibah and Heather were the main two girls that went to the hospital with me and it was important we all agreed to talk to one another about how we felt.

After the fist day I went to visit Maddy in the hospital I wrote her a letter, I wrote it for me just as much as for her; it helped me to process my emotions and tell her how I felt, I have never shown it to her until now, and it reads:

"I have just read your first blog/post and to be honest it practically made me cry, I am so sorry that you are going through all this, you are the last person to ever deserve it!!! And I could only imagine the inner feelings you must be having and the thoughts that are going through your head, but I want you to know that I along with your family, friends and kindly enough over 600 other people are willing to stand by you and with you through this insane journey you have begun. You don't deserve this in the slightest, and the questions that you are faced with are ones that no one should ever have to.

The situation that is before you is unjust and cruel, no one no matter what age but especially this one should have their life torn from beneath them. However, even with the grim riper within sight you still remain bright. You have amazed me with so many things over the very limited but wonderful years that I have known you (#freethenip, #shoesinging) but you have taught me so much more than I could imagine, always stand up for yourself, fight for what you believe in, never take no for an answer. I could probably make a hundred cheesy house quotes from the life lessons that anyone around you long enough would have modelled and taught to them. However, very recently you have taught the whole Facebook community and quite possibly me a very important message, and that is the importance of staying positive.

With all your lessons combined you are fighting cancer the way you go through, you are taking a stand for yourself- inside and out, not taking no for an answer- you're life has only just begun and you will be dammed if it's about to end, fight for what you believe in- fighting for your right to live but on top of all those wonderful Mottos you have added the newest lesson I have learned and that makes you an inspiration and interest to hundreds and that is to always stay positive no matter the situation or to have a crappy house warming hanging always staying "bright no matter how dark the light".

Your ability to handle everything that has come before you, having so much to worry about and reasons to complain, you stay strong. Never once have I heard you say how unfair it is, never once have I heard you ask why me, or state the pain of life's twisted paths. You remain positive and smile. You still laugh and go about life as to not let circumstances bother you. You say FUCK OFF to death and his friends and command your body with the mere will of your soul to stand strong and win the battle within.

It is for this reason and for this reason alone, I believe you have so many eyes upon you, people envy your strength and are in awe of your self-approval, you know you who you are.

You know what you want and you will never apologise for it, an art that in today's society is lost and covered by makeup and money. You are so beautiful, and bright, smart and strong, you put a smile on everyone's face and are taking an unbelievable and approach to all this!! I can only applaud you in the way that you have/had/will conduct your way through this journey but I want you to know that we are all here for you through this whole thing, I know you have heard it hundreds of times, but it is true! And we all love you so much and want nothing but good things. Love you so much darl xx hope you make it through this (I'm sure that you will) xx "

Above all else I want people to recognise that this chapter in anyone's life is difficult, but no matter how hard we as the bystanders think we have it, our friends and loved ones have it a million times harder. Please remember that they are still the same people they always have been, and you will see them in situations that will make you want to cry and feel heartache. They need you, and it is your job to be there for them because you know if the roles were reversed they would do the same. To people who are going through any similar situation, I am so sorry! But it can get better!! If Maddy is a testament to anything it's that you control your body your body doesn't control you, I have seen this first hand, and it can truly amaze. If you are a stranger to this whole life as I was, please do not be afraid, do not ignore it or avoid it because it makes you feel uncomfortable, understand it, know it, help it, and help anyone with going through it in way that you can. And to Maddy, you are honestly the strongest, most powerful self-determined girl I have ever met, I have seen you go through things no one should and the way you have gone about everything will put anyone in awe.   I love you so much and know that you are going to go to great places and this book is just the beginning

Love you always,

Your loyal friend Em xx

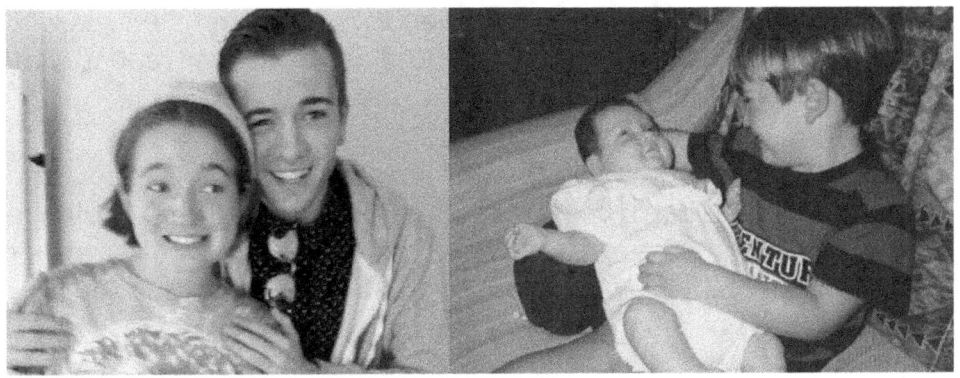

A Sibling's Perspective By Justin Ritchie

To me my sister is the very definition of the word strength. We don't truly know how strong we are until being strong is the only choice we have.

Once cancer happens I believe it changes the way you live and how you look at life and since my sister's diagnosis with Rhabdomyosarcoma I believe it has changed me in a positive light with how I am towards people, my family & friends, my work, my goals & aspirations and how I see the world around me.

I must admit at first, I found it quite difficult to want to accept the fact that this was the cards that we had been dealt and will until this day ask the question as to why my little sister and not me. As an older brother you feel a responsibility and a duty to always protect and look after your younger siblings and in my case Maddy, but when the news of her diagnosis was given to us I suddenly felt like I hadn't done what I'm supposed to do, the feeling as though I was useless and had let her down. I knew from then on that her fight on this journey was mine as well and that I'd be there for her and with her every step of the way, hand in hand.

I knew in myself how much of a beautiful soul my sister is and that for anything to stop her from doing her thing was realistically impossible.

To see my sister for the first time go in for chemotherapy and radiotherapy was hard for me to swallow and a daunting experience for me but what gave me happiness and contentment that things were going to be fine was her smile and amazing attitude towards it all, nothing phases my Mads.

When I am there at the hospital and I see how tired Mads gets and how much of a toll the treatment takes on her body some days, it isn't what any older brother wants to see especially with Mads being only 18, but with that said I'm so happy when I get a text or find out that in the time away from all the hustle and bustle of the hospital she is out most of the time with her friends on weekends, at concerts, seeing a movie with me or just having fun as she should be.

If I had to choose one thing that got me out of bed every morning and motivated me it would be my sister. Despite the long trips up the freeway to Newcastle on a routine basis, all the different medications and procedures that need to be followed, she is always happy, always smiling and willing to do nothing but be active and positive with everything she does. My beautiful mother being the carer for Mads is just as strong a person and knows that together we'll get through all of this one step at a time, together.

The interesting thing about cancer to me is that it's something you never really think about or understand until it happens.

I feel like people tread carefully when they ask or any discussion of the topic arises, and I understand it's not easy and can be awkward. I think it's best to talk about it to people and to make them aware of the situation as well as it being healthy and quite nice to just let people know what I think about it and how it makes me feel.

There are a lot of people out there with great advice and pointers to take from, and there are a lot of people out there where cancer has affected their lives too.

All throughout growing up together, till now and forever I've always seen Mads to be strong, she is a fighter, a warrior, an inspiration and quite frankly there is no other better sister or women out there that could match up or even compare in the slightest, because she is a queen in her own right. We've always been close but I think that this journey has brought us a lot closer and made us realise the important things in life. My sister is clothed with strength and dignity and laughs without fear of the future, and for that, I admire her every day.

Never take a second of life for granted and do whatever makes you happy and most importantly tell those you love every day how much they mean to you.

Justin x

Maddy Ritchie

Chapter Nine

LIFE GOES ON AND CHAKRA POWER

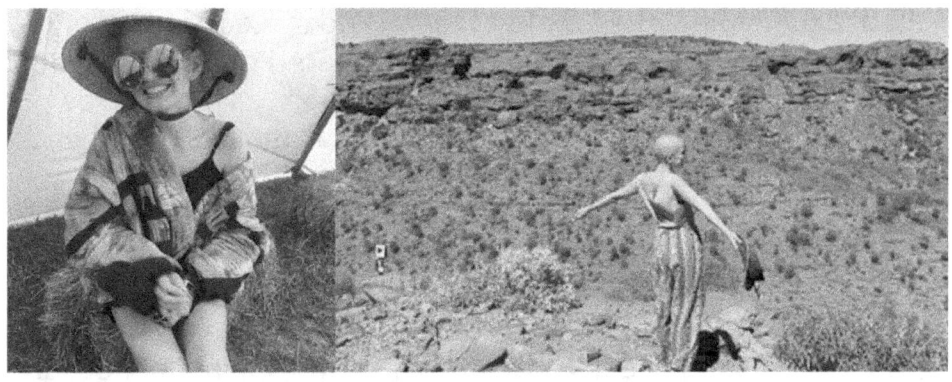

I shared my joyous news of being N.E.D (no evidence of disease) to everyone!

A lot of people assumed my treatment were over and everything was ok, they would say statements of "it must be all over for you in October". In reality, it's not quite like that, yes my treatment and chemotherapy will be over, but the side effects will never be over.

I will have constant check-ups and scans with that 5-year window of will it come back always at the back of my mind. A lot of my life has changed, and I wonder if it will ever truly be the same again.

Dr Frank has told me it could take at least two years for my body to be back to normal and for my energy levels to fully regain.

My fertility will be in limbo until I do IVF at the end of the year and I might not know the full extent until I go to try to have a child of my own. I've also noticed short-term memory loss which is called "chemo brain" as I've become very forgetful especially when my friends reminisce about things.

The thought of getting past 5 years is always at the back of my mind; from prognosis getting to 5 years is below 10% for my cancer.

I choose to not let any of that get to me and make the most of the time I've got whether it is 5 years or 70 years. I don't really know what I'm going to do with myself after October, as I have lived my whole life for the past 11months around hospital stays and visits with no proper routine.

My counsellor says that for teenagers around 18 years it can be very emotional and daunting, as your body hasn't recovered but you want to do something with your life. I'm thinking about doing some sort of course next year, maybe floristry, I'm really not sure.

Throughout my whole cancer period, I always worried about being selfish, but I have learnt it was stupid of me to think like that. It's okay to be selfish when going through cancer or having a very tough time, but I know it's also okay to lean on others.

I have started to go out more recently as treatment has been cut by more than half so I can finally get some of my life back. It is a really lovely feeling to be able to do things somebody my age should be doing.

I struggled the first time walking into a club with people staring and looking at me. After the first time, I honestly couldn't off cared less, just let them stare at your head and think positive thoughts about yourself while they are. It truly doesn't matter what they think.

I've grown apart from some friends and grown closer to the ones that matter the most. The connection I once had with a few of my friends is gone, I struggled with accepting it but they went onto working or University, and it wasn't my world.

I also found that not meeting new people, not working, having a normal routine and feeling somewhat lonely and disconnected from everyone took me to my lowest point; I felt so low it almost made me sick.

Then I found Energy Healing and Chakras!!!!

I had little understanding about Energy Healing and Chakras and didn't understand fully how it works until I met this wonderful lady Naomi. My mum had gone to her for counselling, and she specialised in Women's Health as well as mentoring and energy healing.

One Wednesday evening mum took me along with her to a Women's Group that Naomi was hosting.

At first, I was a bit hesitant as all the women looked at least over 35 years old and were at different stages in their lives. As we went around the room each of them talked about themselves, I went on to learning so much from each of them as they did from me. I felt much empowered by this group and the ladies there, we all talked about stories, current issues we faced and healing. I spoke about my struggles throughout high school and about my diagnosis and how I felt. One lady said she felt very empowered and inspired by my story and another lady felt there was an amazing energy about me.

Naomi felt I had a lot of wisdom and was quite powerful and had this amazing aura around me.

These women helped me to realise my fully value as a woman and human being and also who I am and what I stand for. I learnt about what these women looked back and regretted on and made me realise that having a man around or having kids is not everything.

I walked out feeling really energised and blessed to have had this experience.

A week later mum received a call from Naomi, telling her she had never felt the room feel so powerful; it was something she couldn't explain. Every time I spoke, she found it was very powerful and wanted to explore the aura around me.

She offered to do some healing/body sessions working with chakras with me all free of charge.

Whether religious/spiritual or not, I recommend body works to everyone.

My first session was amazing, I fell into a deep relaxation and felt very at ease. It all has to do with your chakras, balancing and getting rid of blocked energy to create good energy and healing. At first I wasn't quite sure, but in the end, it was the best thing I ever did, it's definitely something you have got to do to believe it.

I walked out from my first session feeling enlightened and balanced, I also learnt that I was no longer alone and that healers and guiders are with me always. Some people have looked at me like I'm a little whacky but once you're there and you're doing it each time the feeling and how you feel the days after are quite astonishing.

I did quite a few sessions with Naomi every fortnight. Each time I developed a better understanding and feel into a deeper state of consciousness and relaxation.

Each time I did it, there was always something new appearing and different parts of my body had blocked energy that needed to be released.

Ever since my first session my journey on learning to heal from my pain and grief has definitely changed for the better. Healing myself, spiritually and mentally couldn't have been done without Naomi and her body healing sessions. I also found talking to her about certain feelings was just an amazing release.

I learnt from these sessions that it's okay to fall apart. As I am now nearing the one-year anniversary of my diagnosis, I can't help but feel pain, grief and sadness. I did get confused with myself at times as I think I should be happy. It's nearly over!

"To let go and move on from your pain and trauma, you need to fall apart. You can't stay strong forever."

-Maddy Ritchie

As I am nearing the one-year anniversary of my diagnosis, I think of the pain, grief and sadness and how far I've come in changing my mindset!

I look back at photos of myself before my diagnosis, and I grieve that girl, I want to go back to looking like the person I was before but I know mentally I've grown into a different person.

I felt like I'd fallen apart and then rebuilt myself, rebuilt my mind to the stronger and improved me. I look towards the better days ahead and to let go of the girl I was before cancer.

The sessions with Naomi immensely helped me mentally and spiritually!

Keep yourself busy and each day for just one minute listen to your breathing and call upon whoever you may believe in or maybe you just want to find healing within yourself and learn to just be. Learn to be happy in your body, learn to heal and to look to the future with positivity.

Feeling guilty is something that I always hear about and is very common among cancer survivors especially young ones. I have not really ever felt that though, in my mind I choose to live for the fighters who have lost their battle with cancer. Everyone in this world serves a purpose, if it wasn't for the ones before me then I don't think I would be here. If it wasn't for the one who dedicated their bodies to cancer research then I don't think I would be here either. If I lost my battle or if cancer ever takes my life I would want the people who won to live out their lives for me.

I definitely respect my fellow cancer survivors for feeling that way, but all I can say is live for them, live your life through the people who have gone before you.

I recently lost a close friend to cancer suddenly. We'd only spoken days before and then she was gone. I had no idea and felt bad, but now I live my life through her and know she is always with me.

I am now coming to the end of my treatment; I only have two more chemos to go. I am physically and mentally exhausted but to make it to the finish line will be such an achievement.

Only time will tell as to how my body will recover from this and we still don't know how affected my leg will be from Vincristine.

Having legs that want to constantly collapse and not walk properly is very frustrating.

I am yet to pull myself together to get my saxophone out from my cupboard, to face the fact that I have mostly if not almost completely forgot those years of learning everything about it are gone from my mind. It might just be a "chemo brain" phase still, and I may regain parts of that memory back with time, but at the moment I can barely remember what note is what and how to play it anymore. I know I will do it soon enough, and re-learn again as I truly have a strong passion for the saxophone. I need more time with facing that, and I will get there.

I have recently met a new guy, I am very attracted to him, and we are dating. We have been going out for a while now, and I've tried to explain to him about my fear and pain if we take it to the next level. He has been very understanding and accepting; we are just taking baby steps at the moment.

The next 5 years of my life will be constantly checking for lumps, bumps and bruises and hoping there will be nothing.

I believe in myself and in my body that I am going to be okay. You can be here one day and gone the next, don't ever let cancer and especially anybody ever control your life.

The power is within you, you have the choice to heal, to live, to love and to learn. You serve a purpose and don't you ever forget that on your journey through life.

My 12-month scan results on the 25th of October 2016 reconfirmed that I am N.E.D and my body no longer had any sort of abnormality. I will stop having treatment altogether now and begin to live again. The day had arrived where I fell to the ground and wept profusely, my torment had finally come to a close, and I made it to the day I had longed to be at for 12 agonising months.

I hope to one day dedicate my life to helping and inspiring others, helping people in need and especially young children and adolescents with cancer.

I also hope to one day create a foundation dedicated to helping the lives of people affected by cancer and their families. I hope to raise the bar on funding for childhood cancer and to create awareness that all cancers should be equal.

I want to help young people connect with others who are going through similar traumas and to help them connect with each other and not feel alone.

I hope this book has helped you as much as it has helped me heal. I want to continue to write more in the future especially about life after cancer and spiritual healing.

If there is a will, there will always be a way. May God be with you all. Thank you.

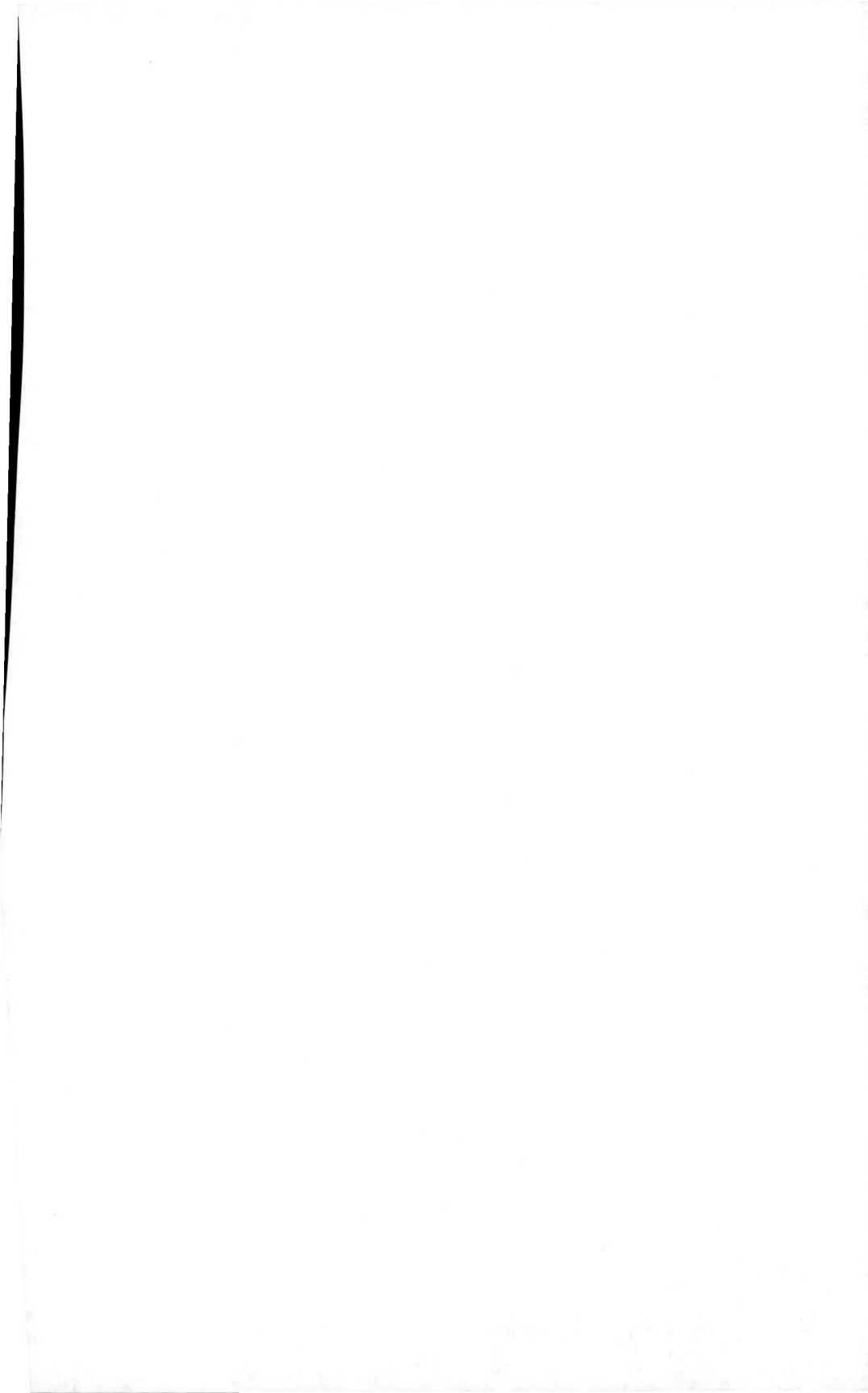

www.ingramcontent.com/pod-product-compliance
Lightning Source LLC
Chambersburg PA
CBHW070146290526
45789CB00002B/649